FLUORIDE
THE
AGING
FACTOR

PARADISE NATURAL FOODS
1868 N. Hillfield Rd. #9
Layton, Utah 84041
(801) 773-3529

FLUORIDE

THE

AGING FACTOR

How to Recognize and Avoid the Devastating Effects of Fluoride

Dr. John Yiamouyiannis

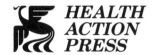

HEALTH ACTION PRESS

International Standard Book Number: 0-913571-03-2
Library of Congress Catalog Card Number: 93-78862

Health Action Press, 6439 Taggart Road, Delaware, Ohio 43015

First edition published 1983
Second edition published 1986
Third edition published 1993

Printed in the United States of America

Cover designed by David Downer and Kevin Lotspaih

"What does it profit my brethren, though a man say he hath faith and have not works? Can faith save him?"

James 2:14

Preface

Tomorrow, BBC-TV will be flying me to London to do a national television program on fluoridation. And CNN is scheduled to do a program on fluoridation after I get back. Why? Well, much has changed since the second edition of this book was published in 1986. And many of the predictions of the first and second editions of this book have now been confirmed.

The *Journal of the American Medical Association* (1990-1992) has reported a greater incidence of hip fractures in fluoridated areas in the U.S. and Britain. The *New England Journal of Medicine* (1990) reported that fluoride treatment of osteoporosis patients resulted in higher hip fracture rates. Government facilities such as Argonne National Laboratories (1988) and the National Institute of Environmental and Health Sciences (1990) have shown that fluoride causes cancer. Former promoters of fluoridation have since found that fluoridation does not reduce tooth decay (1987-1988). In the largest study on fluoridation and tooth decay ever done in the U.S. (1990), it was found that fluoridation is ineffective in reducing tooth decay. Scientists at the U.S. Environmental Protection Agency (1989-1993) have come out against fluoridation because they have confirmed that fluoridation does not reduce tooth decay and that there is clear evidence that fluoridation causes cancer. Animal studies showing fluoride-linked increases in bone cancer and oral cancer have been confirmed by human studies (1991-1993).

The American Chemical Society published a 17-page cover-story questioning the safety and effectiveness of fluoridation (1988). The Rand Corporation has debunked claims by the U.S. Public Health Service that fluoride mouthrinse programs reduce tooth decay (1989-1990). Drinking mineral waters such as Vichy and St. Yorre-Royale has resulted in kidney damage and skeletal fluorosis (1989).

But the real reason for the media attention is that they have become aware of the hype that led to the promotion of this outrageous fraud. And the person responsible for bringing this fraud to their attention was Joel Griffiths. In 1992, Griffiths wrote an article for ***Covert Action*** which gave the media what they had been asking for for years — a motive. He revealed how industries benefited from the promotion of fluoridation. Claims that fluoridation was safe and beneficial to health made it difficult for people to complain when polluting industries belched fluoride out into the air and dumped it into waterways. Such indiscriminate and careless handling of fluoride has allowed companies such as Exxon, U.S. Steel, and ALCOA to make tens of billions of dollars in extra profit at our expense.

In this book, I provide you with the compelling up-to-date evidence showing how fluoridation is chronically poisoning millions. I show why many of the professionals, organizations, and agencies we have relied upon for health information and protection from toxic substances, actually promote the addition of fluoride to public water systems — and why they campaign to stop the removal of fluoride from the drinking water, even in areas where they admit that it is having harmful effects. You get an inside look at the crooked bureaucrats, politicians, and businessmen who profit from human misery. You also get a glimpse at the long list of characters who risked their jobs and careers to get the word out to you that fluoride and fluoridation is taking its toll in human health and life.

Most importantly, I tell you how you can help turn things around and make this world a better place to live.

John Yiamouyiannis
May 29, 1993

Contents

Chapter 1

Speeding Up
The Aging Process

They called it "Das Dorf der jungen Greise", the village where people age before their time. In 1978, the German magazine **Stern** reported on this village of Kizilcaoern, Turkey, describing it as a place where even the young looked and felt old. The article, excerpted here, describes the suffering of these people.

> "The children, the young girls and the only horse in the village have brown teeth. Thirty-year-old men with hunched up shoulders painfully drag themselves around, leaning on sticks. Women produce dead babies after pregnancies of only four months. Forty-year-olds look like old men and women.
>
> "A suspicion that all the villagers could be victims of creeping poisoning was first voiced . . . by a dentist. During a mass examination of children, he discovered a dental disease unknown to him in all children over seven; brown pigmentation on the incisors of the younger children, completely brown teeth in all the older. Adults in the village hardly had any teeth at all. The dentist alerted medical staff at the University Clinic of Eskisehir. Their investigations brought to light even worse news: every single inhabitant of the village suffers from a bone disease—thickening of the ankles, stiffened joints, increased growth of bone substance. The people who live at Kizilcaoern have more bone fractures in arms and legs than other Turks.
>
> "Both men and women suffer from this premature aging. Between 30 and 40, their facial skin becomes wrinkled, muscle tone weakens markedly and they develop walking difficulties.

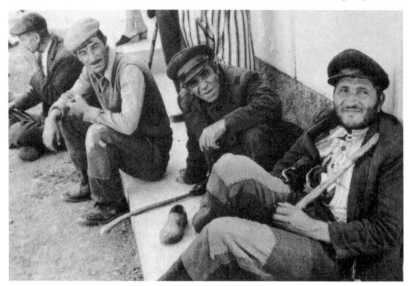

"Even at the age of 30, the residents of Kizilcaoern experience
walking difficulties and wrinkled facial skin. Upon falling, their
bones shatter like glass. Most of them will not reach the age of 50."
[Picture and caption from Stern magazine.]

*"Again and again almost every family has premature
births, with babies stillborn after four or five months of
gestation. Though only 30 years old, one of the men
admits he has lost interest in women. Many of the men
suffer from severe depression because of their early impo-
tence. Most of them do not even enjoy food.*

*"Not even the cattle are in good health. A white-
bearded peasant wearing a black pompom tells of sheep
whose diseased livers after slaughter looked white and
watery.*

*"Dr. Yusuf C. Ozkan as well as his colleagues at the
medical faculty of the University of Eskisehir suspect that
the cause of all this suffering is to be sought in the high
content of fluorides. . . in the neighboring villages which
invariably receive their water from different springs or
wells, the state of health is normal. The medical people
say that the fluoride content of the water is 5.4 parts per
million."*

Similar symptoms have been reported elsewhere. Dr. Frada and co-workers from the University of Palermo reported that the people in the Sicilian village of Acquaviva Platani experienced the same bone and tooth disorders discussed above. They also noticed that these people experience a premature hardening of the arteries and premature senility as well as an increase in mortality which Dr. Frada attributed to the 5 parts per million fluoride found in their drinking water. In India, these fluoride-related bone and tooth disorders have been observed among people drinking water containing fluoride levels as low as 0.7 to 2.5 parts per million. In other areas of India with fluoride levels comparable to those found in Kizilcaoern, the same graphic age-accelerating effects of fluoride can be seen. In 1982, *The Hindu*, India's national newspaper, reported:

> *"In the villages in Dharwar district at Karnataka, a much dreaded disease makes many inhabitants crippled. The naturally high fluorine content in the drinking water sources has led to this affliction and unmitigated suffering which has gone on for a number of years.*
>
> *"A vista of wretchedness unfolds itself as one combs the area for a first-hand study of the magnitude of the problem. The manifestations of the afflictions are clear and in plenty.*
>
> *"The gait, the demeanor, of the menfolk is unusual. There is rigidity in their movements. The early symptom is the discoloration of teeth or what doctors call 'mottling.' With the advancement of age, the teeth fall out giving the appearance of old age, followed by pain in the joints, hips and the loss of flexibility.*
>
> *"'Can you guess my age?' asks Nagappa, a barber by profession, who is in his mid-thirties but looks far beyond fifty."*

Brown teeth, characteristic of the well-known disease, dental fluorosis, has been known in the United States since 1916. Dentists referred to the condition as 'Colorado Brown Stain' and 'Texas Teeth' until 1931, when fluoride in the drinking water was found to be the cause. This disease is now referred to as dental fluorosis. Bone disorders (skeletal fluorosis and osteoporosis and arthritic pains) resulting from fluoride in the drinking water have also been reported in the United States.

In 1943 and 1953 researchers from the United States Public Health Service examined the health status of the residents of Bartlett, Texas to see whether the 8 parts per million fluoride in their drinking water was affecting their health. They found that the mortality rate in Bartlett, Texas was over three times as high as the mortality rate in the neighboring town of Cameron, which contained a much smaller amount of fluoride (0.4 parts per million). While this study examined only a small number of people, the results are supported by data reported by the U.S. Center for Disease Control and the Safe Water Foundation, which indicate that 30,000 to 50,000 excess deaths are observed in the United States each year in areas which add 1 part per million fluoride to the drinking water.

Newburgh, New York was one of the first cities in the United States to be fluoridated. After it was fluoridated in 1945, a number of x-ray examinations were made of the children. In the final report, Dr. John Caffey, a professor of clinical pediatrics at the College of Physicians and Surgeons, Columbia University, noted cortical defects in the bone x-rays of 13.5% of the children living in fluoridated Newburgh, compared to only 7.5% in the neighboring nonfluoridated town of Kingston. The difference was statistically significant and substantive. Dr. Caffey, in another paper, had already reported that these bone defects were strikingly similar to that of osteogenic sarcoma.

It has been known for some time that amounts of fluoride as low as those used to fluoridate public water systems lead to fluoride levels in tissues and organs which damage biologically important chemicals called enzymes. This results in a wide range of chronic diseases.

However, when the results from Kizilcaoern were originally reported, it seemed unlikely that all the symptoms of aging, including premature wrinkling of the skin, could be attributed to the fluoride in the water. It was not until recently that research provided an adequate answer to the following questions:

How could a substance like fluoride cause such aging symptoms as premature skin wrinkling?

Fluoride at levels as low as 1 part per million in the drinking water give rise to an increase in the urine concentration of certain biological chemicals that signal the breakdown of collagen. In addition, fluoride leads to the irregular formation of collagen in the body.

Collagen is important. It makes up 30 percent of the body's protein. The most abundant of all the proteins in the body, it serves as a major structural component of skin, ligaments, tendons, muscles, cartilage, bones and teeth.

Fluoride disruption of this structural protein in skin results in wrinkling. Similarly, fluoride-induced collagen damage results in the weakening of ligaments, tendons, and muscles.

When fluoride induces the breakdown or irregular formation of collagen in cartilage, irreversible arthritis and stiffness of the joints as observed in Kizilcaoern and elsewhere can be expected. Furthermore, fluoride interferes with the production of collagen in cells responsible for laying down tooth enamel and bone. This results in the deformed teeth and bones characteristic of areas with naturally occurring fluoride in the water.

If these startling symptoms of aging were due to fluoride, why haven't such symptoms been found in all the other areas where natural fluoride content in the water is equal to and above that in Kizilcaoern?

As has already been pointed out, these startling aging effects of fluoride have since been found in Italy and India. In these areas, the villagers' poor diet coupled with the relatively high amount of fluoride in their water supply resulted in dramatic aging effects. The villagers' bodies were unable to rebuild the collagen protein that fluoride broke down.

These extreme aging effects occurred among malnourished people drinking water containing fluoride at levels of 5 parts per million. The most important question is:

What is the evidence that fluoride, which is purposely added to the drinking water at a level of 1 part per million, accelerates the aging process even among people consuming the average American diet?

Chapter 2

Symptoms of Fluoride Poisoning in the Western World

To begin to answer, let's refer to the ***United States Pharmacopoeia***, a guide to drug information, which lists some of the side-effects that can result from the daily ingestion of the amount of fluoride found in 1 to 2 pints of artificially fluoridated water. The list includes some of the same symptoms as those mentioned in Chapter 1, as well as allergic-type reactions. (The relationship of these allergic-type reactions to aging will be discussed in Chapter 3.)

Black tarry [tar-like] stools
Bloody vomit
Faintness
Nausea and vomiting
Shallow breathing
Stomach cramps or pain
Tremors
Unusual excitement
Unusual increase in saliva
Watery eyes
Weakness
Constipation
Loss of appetite
Pain and aching of bones
Skin rash
Sores in the mouth and on the lips
Stiffness
Weight loss
White, brown, or black discoloration of teeth

According to the **U.S. Pharmacopoeia**: *"Although not all of these side-effects appear very often, when they do occur they may require medical attention."*

The **1991 Physicians' Desk Reference** cautions: *"Dental fluorosis [mottling] may result from exceeding the recommended dose. In hypersensitive individuals, fluorides occasionally cause skin eruptions such as atopic dermatitis, eczema, or urticaria. Gastric distress, headache, and weakness have also been reported. These hypersensitive reactions usually disappear promptly after discontinuation of the fluoride. In rare cases, a delay in the eruption of teeth has been reported."*

Some people drink more water. When asked about diabetics, Kathy Krausfelder from the National Institutes of Arthritis, Diabetes and Digestive and Kidney Disease stated: *"The symptoms of diabetes include rapid weight loss, excessive thirst, frequent urination"* and pointed out that: *"According to the National Institute of Dental Research, . . . fluoride levels in water are set according to normal consumption of water. If an individual is consuming abnormally large quantities of water, he should drink bottled water."*

Well, as a matter of fact, **many American physicians have observed these fluoride-induced diseases in their everyday practices even among people consuming normal quantities**.

Dr. William P. Murphy, who won the Nobel Prize for his research which led to the cure of pernicious anemia, is among those who have observed the adverse effects of fluoride.

He recounts a patient of his who *"while living in a community in which the water was fluoridated had rather continuous swelling of the lower legs and face, aggravated by certain foods or medications to which she was allergic. After moving from this community to a non-fluoridated one this swelling largely disappeared and only appears now after exposure to fairly large amounts of allergens. After moving she started using a fluoride toothpaste at which time she developed a rash on her cheeks and mouth with swelling of the face. After stopping this toothpaste this condition cleared up completely."*

The following is an account of a 62-year-old patient examined by Dr. C.D. Marsh of Memphis, Tennessee: The woman lived in Memphis which was not fluoridated at that time. Whenever she traveled to Washington D.C. and Richmond, Virginia — both fluoridated cities — she invariably developed excruciating abdominal pain, headache, backache, and profuse nasal discharge, followed by diarrhea and lethargy. These symptoms disappeared promptly within a few days after her return home. She avoided these problems on future trips to the two cities by taking several bottles of Memphis water with her and avoiding fluid foods. Then twice she came down with the illness, to her surprise, while at home. Dr. Marsh traced these reoccurrences to a fluorine-containing tranquilizer (trifluoperazine) prescribed by him and, on the other occasion, to a fluoridated toothpaste. A double-blind test carried out by Dr. Marsh confirmed fluoride as the cause of the illness.

Dr. John J. Shea of Dayton, Ohio relates one of his experiences: *"Mr. E.H., age 48, consulted. . .[me] because of giant urticaria [itchy red skin eruptions] of one month's duration. The lesions involved mainly hands and feet and at times the entire body surface. At the first visit the lips and gums showed a marked edema [swelling]. The lesions usually occurred about one hour after breakfast. The patient had been using a fluoride toothpaste at that time.*

"He was asked to discontinue the fluoride toothpaste and not to take any medication. Three days later, he reported having had only a single hive and slight residual pruritus [itching]. Six days later, he was completely free of symptoms. Three years later, this patient experienced another episode of generalized urticaria. In the morning he had inadvertently brushed his teeth with a toothpaste used by his family without realizing that it was a fluoride brand. The hives appeared within one hour of its use."

Dr. S.M. Gillespie relates the following: *"C.E.O., a seven-month-old female child, had been taking Tri-Vi-Flor [vitamin drops with fluoride] daily for five weeks. About that time she developed an exudative, pruritic dermatitis [itchy red skin eruptions] on the neck, face and in the antecubital and retropopliteal areas [arms and legs] accompanied by diarrhea, abdominal cramps and bloody stool. The parents noted that the cramps occurred exclusively, shortly after the afternoon feedings when the baby received fluoride drops. The drug, therefore, was discontinued. The skin immediately began to clear up. Within one week the eruption had healed, no medication had been prescribed. The child has been in good health ever since."*

Dr. G.W. Grimbergen and a group of Dutch physicians studied 60 patients suffering from diseases induced by fluoride in the drinking water. Fifty percent suffered gastrointestinal disorders, 25 percent suffered from inflammatory diseases involving the mouth, 8 percent experienced excessive thirst, 5 percent experienced joint pains and/or migraine headaches and/or visual disturbances, and 3 percent experienced a ringing sensation in the ears and/or mental depression.

Dr. Jonathan Forman, an allergist from Columbus, Ohio relates: *"In our own practice, we have run down cases of hives, behavior problems, and several patients which others had labeled neurotics to be due to fluoride intoxication."* He pointed out that when these people were put on distilled water and when fluorine-containing foods were removed from their diet, they recovered. When fluorine was introduced back into their diets, their symptoms returned.

Drs. Luis Juncos and James Donadio of the Mayo Clinic described a 17-year-old girl and an 18-year old boy who had skeletal and dental fluorosis, accompanied by markedly reduced kidney function. The youths' primary source of drinking water contained 1.7 and 2.6 parts per million fluoride, respectively. In regard to these two cases, Drs. Juncos and Donadio concluded that either fluoride was damaging the kidney or that fluoride was not being removed from the body because of an already damaged kidney. The possibility that fluoride damaged the kidneys in these cases is supported by evidence from the Yerkes Primate Research Center in Atlanta and Cornell University which show that 1 to 5 parts per million fluoride causes interference with enzymes in the kidney and kidney damage in laboratory animals.

Dr. George Waldbott of Warren, Michigan observed fluoride-induced diseases in over 400 cases of fluoride exposure. One of his most severe cases was a 35-year-old woman from Highland

Park, Michigan, which was fluoridated at that time. Dr. Waldbott recorded her symptoms as follows: *"She was constantly nauseated, vomited frequently, had sharp epigastric [abdominal] pain and diarrhea, and complained of pain in the lower back.*

"She reported progressive weight loss, had repeated hematuria [bloody urine], uterine hemorrhages, and constant pain throughout her head. Her eyesight had gradually deteriorated. She had noticed scotomas [blind spots] in both eyes and lesions on the arms and legs. Weakness in the hands and arms prevented grasping certain objects. Furthermore, due to loss of control of legs and lack of coordination of her thoughts she eventually became incoherent, drowsy, and forgetful."

Her health deteriorated further, forcing her to a bedridden state. She was hospitalized for diagnostic tests. Nine specialists were unable to determine the cause of her disease.

"After the tests were completed, she began drinking unfluoridated . . . water. Within two days the gastrointestinal symptoms and headaches subsided without medication, and she was soon well enough to be discharged.

"At home she strictly avoided fluoridated water for drinking as well as for cooking her food and avoided . . . [food with a] high fluoride content. The headaches, eye disturbances, and muscular weaknesses disappeared in a most dramatic manner. After about two weeks her mind began to clear, and she had a complete change in personality. In subsequent tests, each time she was given fluoride, her symptoms returned."

Dr. Waldbott has also observed fluoride-induced diseases among people living near fluoride-emitting factories (e.g., aluminum, phosphate, steel, and frit [frit is the glassy substance used to coat the inside of ovens] manufacturers) as well as in workers employed in these industries. The major complaints he found in the 133 cases which he examined were arthritis, respiratory problems, gastrointestinal disorders, and headaches along with other neurological complications.

In 1977, Dr. Bertram Carnow, Professor and Director of Occupational and Environmental Medicine of the University of Illinois School of Public Health and Director of the Division of Occupational Medicine of the Cook County Hospital, and Dr.

Shirley Conibear, Director of the Health Hazards Unit of the Cook County Hospital, studied the health status of 1242 aluminum workers exposed to airborne fluorides. They reported:

"A highly significant relationship was found between increasing levels of exposure to fluorides and other pulmonary irritants and obstructive pulmonary changes."

They pointed out that measurements showing these obstructive changes suggested a *"decreased elasticity of the lungs"*. They cited the finding of other investigators that fluoride induced pulmonary fibrosis, i.e. increased levels of collagen in the lung.

Drs. Carnow and Conibear also found that increasing levels of exposure to fluoride were related to arthritis and back pains, as observed in Kizilcaoern and Karnataka (see Chapter 1), and reported their results as follows:

Worker Exposure	Workers with Musculoskeletal Problems (Mostly Arthritis and Back Problems)
Low	30.2%
Medium	32.1%
Medium-High	41.8%
High	52.0%

In their recommendations they state:

"Given this study's findings of pulmonary and musculoskeletal disease, even among those only moderately exposed, it would seem that a major effort should be made immediately to reduce the levels of irritant gases (hydrogen fluoride) and particulate (fluoride salts)."

In a survey of 370 aluminum potroom workers in western Norway, increased prevalences of respiratory symptoms, work-related asthmatic symptoms, and abnormal lung function were found in subjects exposed to higher fluoride levels in the air when compared with workers exposed to lower levels of fluoride. In Russia, 378 workers in an aluminum plant were found with calcified ligaments and abnormal bony outgrowths as a result of fluoride exposure. Eighty-five per cent of these workers experienced bone and joint pains.

The health hazards of airborne fluorides from industry have been known for a long time and have been reported by many investigators. The main symptoms reported are rheumatic pains, respiratory disorders, nausea and loss of appetite. Those reporting fluoride-induced diseases among people living near fluoride-polluting industries include Dr. M. Klotz from West Germany and Drs. M.M. Murray and D.C. Wilson from England. Still more have found fluoride-induced diseases among factory workers exposed to high levels of fluoride. These include Dr. Kaj Roholm from Denmark, Dr. E. Speder from France, Dr. H.H. Schlegel from Switzerland, and Dr. J. Franke from East Germany.

Mass poisonings from fluoride emissions from aluminum, phosphate, and other industries have been reported in Maryland, Florida, Quebec, Ohio, Oregon, Washington, and British Columbia, as well as in other places. In an air pollution disaster in Donora, Pennsylvania, 20 people lost their lives with lethal levels of fluoride in their blood. In another incident in the Belgian Meuse Valley, 60 persons lost their lives. In Spencer County, Indiana, population 18,000, 79 persons living around a fluoride polluting plant died between January 1 and May 31, 1978, many of them from a disease called 'sudden death syndrome'. The coroner is convinced that fluoride emissions from the local aluminum plant were to blame.

Excessive discharges of fluoride into the air are not the only means by which people can be exposed to lethal doses of fluoride.

Acute Fluoride Poisoning

Make no mistake about it, fluoride is a poison. According to the 1984 issue of *Clinical Toxicology of Commercial Products* (Williams & Wilkins), it is more poisonous than lead and just slightly less poisonous than arsenic. It has been used as a pesticide for the control of mice, rats, and other small pests. In 1991, the Akron (Ohio) Regional Poison Center reported that *"Death has been reported following ingestion of 16 mg/kg of fluoride."* In English that we can all understand, that means that one-hundreth of an ounce of fluoride could kill a 10-pound child and one-tenth of an ounce could kill a 100-pound adult.

The Akron Regional Poison Center continues *"Fluoride tooth-paste contains up to 1 mg/gram of fluoride."* This means that a family-sized tube of toothpaste contains 199 milligrams of fluoride, more than enough to kill a 25-pound child. Even Procter and Gamble, the makers of Crest, acknowledges that a family-sized (7-ounce) tube of fluoride toothpaste *"theoretically, at least, contains enough fluoride to kill a small child."*

While most children will not consume an entire tube of toothpaste, consumption of smaller amounts of toothpaste certainly presents a health hazard.

The toothbrushing habits of 12- to 24-month-old children were examined and it was found that 20% of the children ingested more than 0.25 mg of fluoride per day by toothbrushing alone. It has been found that a 4- to 6-year-old child will consume 25% to 33% of the toothpaste on their brush. Swedish scientists, concerned about this added intake, issued the following warning: if pre-school children living in a naturally fluoridated area (artificial fluoridation has been banned in Sweden) brush their teeth with fluoridated toothpaste, they should only be allowed to brush their teeth once a day, and then only with a pea-sized amount of toothpaste under the supervision of an adult.

Eighty-seven cases of fluoride poisonings in children younger than 12 years old were reported to the Rocky Mountain Poison Control Center in 1986. Eighty-five cases involved accidental ingestion of fluoride products in the home. Two involved fluoride treatment by a dentist. One 13-month-old child died. Twenty-five suffered gastrointestinal symptoms (nausea, vomiting, diarrhea, abdominal pain). In a more recent study, it was reported that sodium fluoride, the same type used in Crest toothpaste, was the most frequent single cause of acute poisoning in children.

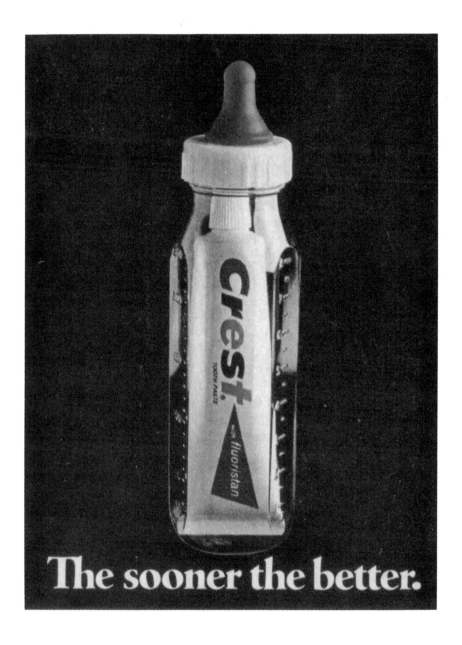

This ad has appeared in widely read magazines such as *Reader's Digest* and *Redbook*.

The Annapolis Spill

On November 11, 1979, up to 50 parts per million fluoride was dumped into the Annapolis, Maryland public water system. This resulted in the poisoning of 50,000 people. At the request of the local newspaper, the ***Annapolis Evening Capital***, Dr. Yiamouyiannis went to Annapolis to investigate the damage that had been done. He conducted an epidemiological study and found that approximately 10,000 people exhibited acute symptoms of fluoride poisoning. His findings were subsequently confirmed by the Maryland State Department of Health. While the Maryland Department of Health refused to disclose the number of citizens who died of heart failure due to the spill, Dr. Yiamouyiannis found that more than five times the normal number of people died of heart failure during the week following the spill.

Dr. Yiamouyiannis enlisted the aid of Dr. Waldbott who conducted a clinical survey of people in the Annapolis area. Dr. Waldbott interviewed 112 persons who believed they had suffered adverse reactions from the spill. He recorded the presence or absence of known symptoms of fluoride poisoning. Of the 112 interviewed, 103 were diagnosed as suffering from fluoride poisoning; of the 103, 62% complained of musculoskeletal symptoms, 65% neurological symptoms, 81% gastrointestinal symptoms, 59% urological symptoms, and 13% dermatological symptoms. These results confirmed already-reported information about fluoride intoxication from drinking water. [The Annapolis spill is not an isolated case. For more information about other fluoride spills, see Appendix.]

Even fluoridated bottled water can be fatal. On March 30, 1989, the California Department of Health Services reported that Niagara brand bottled water was found to contain 450 parts per million fluoride. State health director Kenneth Kizer warned that *"Consumption of these high levels of fluoride in water could produce stomachache, nausea, vomiting, serious illness, or even death."*

Lethal Overdoses in the Dental Chair

On January 20, 1979, the **New York Times** ran the following story:

$750,000 Given in Child's Death in Fluoride Case— Boy, 3, Was in City Clinic for Routine Cleaning

"A State Supreme Court jury awarded $750,000 to the parents of a 3-year-old Brooklyn boy who, on his first trip to the dentist in 1974, was given a lethal dose of fluoride at a city dental clinic and then ignored for nearly five hours in the waiting rooms of a pediatric clinic and Brookdale Hospital while his mother pleaded for help, and he lapsed into a coma and died.

"Mrs. Kennerly testified that she took William, born on Feb. 7, 1971, for his first dental checkup on May 24, 1974 to the Brownsville Dental Health Center, a city clinic at 259 Bristol Street.

"There, he was examined by Dr. George, who found no dental caries and turned the boy over to Miss Cohen, a dental hygienist, for routine teeth-cleaning. After cleaning William's teeth, witnesses explained, Miss Cohen, using a swab, spread a stannous fluoride jell over the boy's teeth as a decay-preventive.

"According to Mrs. Kennerly, Miss Cohen was engrossed in conversation while working on William and, after handing him a cup of water, failed to instruct him to wash his mouth out and spit out the solution. Mrs. Kennerly said William drank the water.

"According to a Nassau County toxicologist, Dr. Jesse Bidanset, William ingested 45 cubic centimeters of 2 percent stannous fluoride solution, triple an amount sufficient to have been fatal.

"William began vomiting, sweating and complaining of headache and dizziness. His mother, appealing to the dentist, was told the child had been given only a routine treatment. But she was not satisfied, and was sent to the Brookdale Ambulatory Pediatric Care Unit in the same

building.

"Mrs. Kennerly testified that she had waited there two and a half hours, appealing for help, as her son became progressively more sick, lapsing into what she thought was sleep, but actually was a coma.

"Finally taken into an examination room, the boy was seen by Dr. Bathia, who summoned a supervisor. They injected adrenalin into the boy's heart to revive him. An ambulance took him to Brookdale Hospital, a five-minute drive away.

"There, William and his mother waited more than an hour. By then, he had lapsed back into a coma, and as doctors attempted to pump his stomach, he went into cardiac arrest, and died at 2:10 p.m."

Terry Leder, a dental hygienist from Glen Cove, Long Island witnessed a similar tragedy in 1969. At the time she worked in a New York City dental clinic.

"One of my bosses was working on a patient and applied topical fluoride," Ms. Leder recalled in a recorded interview in 1979. *"The child went into convulsions and died in the chair. We were all shocked. It happened so fast that nobody could do anything for him. It was just a few minutes after the fluoride was applied."*

The clinic, claiming the child died of a heart attack even though he had no history of heart problems, denied any responsibility for the death. Ms. Leder pointed out that the parents *"never got the true answer"*.

She now refuses to apply fluoride to a patient's teeth.

"I just feel it's very dangerous for the safety of my kids. And I feel that they're my kids. Anybody who comes into my office, in my chair, belongs to me while they're there. I won't do anything to hurt them." Ms. Leder added that the dentist she works for trusts her and allows her to have a free hand.

Ms. Leder outlined the typical fluoride treatment. She pointed out that 10,000 parts per million fluoride (which comes in flavors to make it more palatable) is left on the teeth for about five minutes. Then the child spits it out, though invariably he/she swallows some. The child cannot rinse, eat or drink for at least a half hour afterwards to let the fluoride soak into the teeth.

Some parents, she said, report that their children become nauseous after fluoride treatments; they still want the fluoride administered, though, because they believe it will reduce tooth decay and lower their dental costs.

After researching the matter, Ms. Leder isn't convinced that fluoride does in fact reduce or prevent tooth decay. *"I just wish parents would read before they subject their children to something so dangerous"*, she said. *"It's not going to save money. Good oral hygiene is going to prevent tooth decay. Fluoride isn't."* [According to N.C. Cons of the New York State Bureau of Dental Health, and Dr. Herschel S. Horowitz of the U.S. Public Health Service, topical fluoride is practically ineffective in reducing tooth decay. Additional warnings of danger to gum tissues and dentinal tubules were voiced at the American Association for the Advancement of Science as long ago as 1977 where it was pointed out that: *"There should be continuing concern and control with fluorides in all forms that are now becoming individually administered for home care (tablet, mouthwash, gels, toothpaste, etc.). The high concentrations of some products may be neither biologically desirable nor clinically necessary."*]

On July 21, 1990, Chuck Filippini took his 8-year-old daughter to the dentist and received a fluoride treatment at 11:00 A.M. Two hours later, she went into a seizure. Two to three days later, she died.

These cases aren't unusual. Surveys show that over 6% of the children receiving fluoride treatments at the dental office complained of side-effects, including nausea and vomiting, either immediately or within one hour following treatment.

Other Acute Reactions

Dr. Milton A. Saunders, a physician from Virginia Beach, Virginia, reported that acne-like eruptions also result from the mere contact of fluoridated toothpaste with areas around the mouth. In his report, published in ***Archives of Dermatology***, he noted: *"I requested that these patients switch, on a trial basis,*

from their fluoride toothpastes to a nonfluoride toothpaste.
Within a period varying from two to four weeks, approximately
one half the patients thus observed cleared of their previously
persistent acne-like eruption. Several of the patients, who were
concerned about the dental health factors relative to fluoride and
its exclusion, requested to resume use of a fluoride toothpaste.
These patients were then allowed to resume use of a fluoride
toothpaste. Without exception, each developed the same distribu-
tion of acne-like eruption that had previously occurred."

The findings of Dr. Saunders have since been corroborated
by Dr. J. Ramsey Mellette and co-workers of the United States
Army who *"have gathered clinical and historical data implicat-*
ing fluoride dentifrices as an important etiologic factor in the
dermatosis."

On November 3, 1979, the ***Melbourne Truth*** of Australia
carried the following story:

Fluoride Tablets Kill Baby Jason

"Jason lapsed into a coma and died five days later at the
Mater Children's Hospital in South Brisbane.
   "A spokesman for the Queensland Justice Department
confirmed that Jason's death was caused by fluoride
poisoning. He said the death certificate was authentic. It
records the cause of death as fluoride poisoning.
   "Mrs. Burton [Jason's mother] recalled the day her
nightmare began: 'I was getting some carpet laid while
Jason was having his afternoon sleep. After about five
minutes—definitely not more than seven—I got the feeling
something was the matter. Jason was sitting on the floor
with a bottle of fluoride tablets. I rang the doctor and said
Jason had taken some of the tablets, not many . . . about
half a dozen.
   "Mrs. Burton said the doctor told her to take Jason
down to him and had then given the child a stomach
pump. 'I asked the doctor if he had found any fluoride
tablets and he replied that he had found four.'
   "Later, Mrs. Burton found her son had become uncon-
scious. She took him to the hospital. She said a tube was
placed in her son's throat and he was connected to a

respirator.

"Four days later, a brain specialist examined Jason and told Mrs. Burton her son was technically but not yet clinically dead. The next day, according to Mrs. Burton, the life support system was removed and Jason died.

"She said: 'They (the doctors) told me at first that it was impossible for fluoride to kill my son. Finally they said that it was the fluoride.'

"Mrs. Burton said Jason had been taking fluoride tablets every day since his first birthday. In addition, she had been told to take them during her pregnancy."

How many child deaths from 'sudden infant death syndrome' are associated with the consumption of or overdose of fluoride from tablets, toothpastes, and dental treatments? This is still hard to determine. Even in the above three cases, where it was clearly shown that these childhood diseases were due to fluoride, the attending physicians and dentists refused to admit openly that fluoride was the killer. Think how much harder it is to recognize fluoride as the villain when it works more slowly as in the following case related by Cynthia Markos of Battle Creek, Michigan:

"It all started when my 5-year-old son, Eric Markos, was given fluoride rinses weekly at the Head Start Program. Naturally, I signed a permission slip for him to participate in the program; I was always led to believe fluoride is great. No one from the Head Start Program informed me that it could cause problems for children.

"Eric started the Head Start Program on October 14, 1980. The fluoride rinsing started the week of October 20th, 1980. By Thanksgiving, November 26, 1980, Eric was having stomach aches once-twice a week. His appetite was not like it had been, he was always tired and wanted to sleep a lot. One of his teachers informed me that he was sick quite often at school and had to lie down. She said he would sometimes turn pale in the face when he complained of stomach aches. His problem seemed to get worse, more severe pain on the weekends. Finally, on February 20, 1981, I took Eric to see his pediatrician, Dr.

*Joseph Levy. Dr. Levy examined Eric in his office as
thoroughly as possible. He also gave Eric a Pin Worm
test, which turned out to be negative. The doctor thought
it was possibly his nerves doing this. As Eric's mother I
didn't go along with this theory at all. Dr. Levy could find
no physical problems with Eric. Eric continued having
stomach problems, loss of appetite, and fatigue.*

*"On March 17, 1981 I met Mr. Andrew Craig. He got
on the subject of fluoridated water in the city of Battle
Creek. He made a statement which really hit home with
me. 'Fluoride is a poison and can cause, in small children
especially, gastrointestinal tract problems.' After talking
with Mr. Craig about fluoride, I informed him of my son's
problems and that he was on a fluoride rinse program.
He then gave me quite a bit of information pertaining to
fluoride. After reading all of the information and thinking back about when Eric's problems started I decided
this could be the cause of his stomach aches. So I took
Eric completely off the rinse program, fluoridated toothpaste at home, and all natural fluoride food and drinks.*

*"Well, Eric's health was 100% better after just one
week of being off the fluoride. I look back now and realize
how sick Eric really was. Seeing him healthy now is such
a great a relief I don't want to think about what could
have happened to him if we hadn't caught the fluoride
overfeed in time."*

Fluoride mouth-rinse programs are currently being administered to children by teachers. Since these teachers are not
licensed to practice medicine, dentistry, or pharmacy, fluoride
mouth-rinse programs are illegal. To administer the drug,
teachers are required to take 3- to 4-gram packets of sodium
fluoride (enough to kill 3 to 6 children) and dilute them for use
by the children. This is in violation of pharmacy laws which
prohibit the compounding or dispensing of drugs without a
license. Fluoride is classified both as a drug and as a poison.
Furthermore, in the administration of this program to students,
the teacher, as well as the school board, are guilty of practicing
medicine without a license. Additionally, since most school rinse

programs do not make the parent aware of the warning on the fluoride rinse packets, "AMOUNT IS POISONOUS IF SWALLOWED. KEEP AWAY FROM CHILDREN." and "WARNING: DO NOT SWALLOW", they are in violation of laws requiring the terminal distributor to make the parents aware of the danger involved.

Tide Beginning to Turn?

Even the promoters of fluoridation and the fluoride supplements are beginning to leave the ship, but as they delay, they continue to subject the innocent, trusting, and unaware public to the devastating effects of fluoride. Consider the following:

In 1977, the *Fluoride Symposium of the 143rd Annual meeting of the American Association for the Advancement of Science* and again in 1978, the *Journal of the American Dental Association* reported that 0.5 mg fluoride supplements were causing dental fluorosis. But nothing was done about it and millions of children have been poisoned as a result.

In the *1978 Physicians' Desk Reference* (p. 1637), the following statement with regard to fluoride supplements was made: *"A daily fluoride intake of 0.5 mg. from birth to age three years . . . is recommended."*

Then, in the *1983 Physicians' Desk Reference* (p. 1977), the following statement with regard to fluoride supplements was made: *"In communities with less than 0.3 ppm fluoride in the water supply, the recommended dosage is 0.25 mg daily between birth and two years of age."* The recommended dose had been cut in half.

Finally, in the 1992 Canadian Dental Association Proposed Fluoride Guidelines, the following statement was made: *"Fluoride supplements should not be recommended for children less than three years old."*

In 1993, thanks to the tenacity of a New Jersey legislative aide, Michael Perrone, the FDA was forced to admit: (1) that they have no studies showing that fluoride tablets or drops are either safe or effective in reducing tooth decay and (2) that the sale of fluoride tablets and drops is illegal. If it acts responsibly, the

FDA (which admitted that legally, fluoride tablets and drops should be removed from the market) will take fluoride tablets and drops off the market before this book gets off the press.

Discussion of Clinical Findings

It is difficult, in these clinical observations, to determine the exact mechanism of fluoride action. The skin diseases could be the result of fluoride inducing the distortion of body proteins (see Chapters 3, 4, and 11), which, not recognized by the body, induces the body's immune system to attack it.

The arthritic symptoms of back pains, stiffness, and aching bones could be a mild form of the fluoride-induced osteoarthritis observed in Kizilcaoern, Turkey as well as in India (see Chapter 1). Alternatively, these symptoms could be rheumatoid arthritis brought about by an autoimmune response to the fluoride-induced production of imperfect collagen in bone, cartilage, ligaments, and/or tendons.

The gastrointestinal symptoms result from the direct toxic effects of fluoride on the stomach and the inhibition of intestinal bacteria. These bacteria aid in the digestion of food and when they are inhibited, gastrointestinal disorders can be expected.

The symptom of fatigue is probably the result of the inhibitory effect of fluoride on thyroid activity. As pointed out by the **Merck Index**, fluoride was formerly used to depress thyroid activity. As little as 5 milligrams, the amount consumed daily by people drinking fluoridated water, has been shown to lower thyroid activity in humans.

In rare cases, immediate death from fluoride occurs as a result of cardiac arrest, possibly brought on in some cases by an anaphylactic (or anaphylactoid) shock. More often, fluoride-induced acceleration of the aging process leads to disease so persistently severe that death is an eventual, though not immediate result.

WARNING: Everyone being exposed to the levels of
fluoride found in the fluoridated drinking water is being
chronically poisoned. Recurrent 'upset stomachs', arthritis, skin problems, weakness, etc. are diseases which
people begin to accept as normal. As these diseases
become more severe, they are attributed to 'old age'. Of
special interest is the fact that before any disease is even
noticeable, the acceleration of the aging process by
fluoride is already occurring at the biochemical level (by
means of enzyme inhibition, collagen breakdown, genetic damage, and/or disruption of the immune system
per se). People who do not experience one or more of the
overt fluoride-induced clinical symptoms will invariably
be experiencing the fluoride-induced subclinical deterioration of the body commonly referred to as aging.

Chapter 3

Disarming the Immune System

The immune system is the body's major defense mechanism against disease. It is composed of white blood cells and a number of tissues throughout the body that make or activate white blood cells. These cells serve as the body's surveillance system to recognize and destroy foreign agents such as bacteria, viruses, and chemicals as well as the body's own obsolete, damaged, or cancerous cells.

When the immune system is working optimally, infections are stopped quickly and the disease is 'nipped in the bud'.

As people age, their immune system becomes less able to recognize the difference between the agents that it should attack and the component cells or cell products of their own body. This may result in an 'autoimmune' allergic response. (An autoimmune response is a process in which the immune system begins to attack and destroy the body's own tissue.) In such cases, the clinical observations of skin rashes, gastrointestinal disorders, etc., which are common among the elderly, will result. Many scientists believe that the cumulative effect of tissue damage by the autoimmune response is a major factor in the aging process.

Even when white blood cells properly recognize the agents they should be attacking, the speed with which white cells get to these agents and destroy them diminishes with age. As a result, the body's ability to fight infections is retarded and the 'elderly' patient suffers much more severe diseases — some even leading to death — than their 'younger' counterparts, who, when challenged with the same infections, suffer little if any discomfort.

Tricking the Immune System

In 1981, Dr. John Emsley and co-workers at King's College in London found that fluoride strongly interacts with forces (or bonds) which maintain the normal shapes of different proteins in the body. The ability of fluoride to interfere with the normal shape and function of proteins has since been confirmed by Dr. Steven Edwards and co-workers from the University of California at San Diego and Drs. H.C. Froede and I.B. Wilson from the University of Colorado at Boulder. By distorting the conformation of the body's own protein, the immune system attacks its own protein resulting in the autoimmune or allergic response described in Chapter 2.

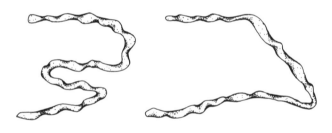

Normal Protein   **Distorted Protein**

Damaging the Immune System

In order for white blood cells to get to the agent that they must destroy, they must first be passively carried to the general area through the bloodstream. At that point, they must squeeze through the walls of blood vessels and literally 'creep' through to the location of the agent to be destroyed.

Dr. Peter Wilkinson of the University of Glasgow found that fluoride decreased the migration rate of human white blood cells. He used a chemical (called a chemotactic agent) to attract

the white blood cells, but obstructed their movement by putting
a filter in their way. This forced the white blood cells to squeeze
their way through the filter in an attempt to reach the chemotactic agent. (Chemotactic agents are substances released by
foreign invaders to the body. These chemotactic agents signal
the white blood cells to get to and destroy the foreign invaders.)
He then measured the distance traveled by these white blood
cells into the filter.

 The following table shows the migration rates of white blood
cells treated with various concentrations of fluoride for 30
minutes relative to white cells not treated with fluoride. As can
be seen from this table, as little as 0.2 part per million fluoride,
the amount of fluoride found in the blood of people living in
fluoridated areas, inhibited the movement of white cells. As the
fluoride concentration increased, so did the degree of migration
inhibition.

THE EFFECT OF FLUORIDE ON THE MIGRATION OF WHITE BLOOD CELLS

Fluoride Concentration	Exposure Time	Relative Migration Rate
0 ppm	30 minutes	100%
.2 ppm	30 minutes	92%
2 ppm	30 minutes	85%
20 ppm	30 minutes	65%
200 ppm	30 minutes	0%

Dr. Sheila Gibson used blood samples from 100 different people
and looked at unobstructed migration of white blood cells for
each of the 100 samples. Taking an average of all the samples,
she showed that fluoride decreased the migration rate of human
white blood cells at a rate comparable to the results obtained by
Wilkinson.

THE EFFECT OF FLUORIDE ON THE MIGRATION OF WHITE BLOOD CELLS

Fluoride Concentration	Exposure Time	Relative Migration Rate
0 ppm	3 hours	100%
.5 ppm	3 hours	91%
1 ppm	3 hours	89%
2 ppm	3 hours	84%
20 ppm	3 hours	73%

Although these studies were done using human white blood cells, they are what might be termed test-tube experiments. What happens, for example, when 1 part per million fluoride is consumed through the drinking water?

The Effect of Fluoride on Cyclic AMP

Dr. D.W. Allman and co-workers from the Indiana University School of Medicine fed animals 1 part per million fluoride and noticed that urinary levels of a substance made in the body called cyclic AMP (adenosine monophosphate) increased by more than 100%. They also found comparable increases in cyclic AMP levels in the body's soft tissues. More recently they found that, in the presence of aluminum, as little as 20-100 parts per <u>billion</u> fluoride is able to cause an increase in cyclic AMP levels.

These findings are significant because cyclic AMP inhibits the migration rate of white blood cells (as shown by Dr. Israel Rivkin and co-workers from the University of Minnesota, and others), as well as the ability of white blood cells to destroy foreign agents such as bacteria, viruses, etc. (as shown by Dr. Gerald Weissmann and co-workers from the New York University School of Medicine, and others).

Dr. J. Gabrovsek, a research dentist at Case Western Reserve University School of Medicine, recognized the significance of the effects of fluoride-induced increases in cyclic AMP levels and the effect that this might have on the immune system. In

1980, he published a paper, stating:

"Because of the inhibitory effects of NaF [sodium fluoride] on phagocytosis and leukotaxis (the migration of white blood cells), which are basic defense mechanisms, I have doubts about the absolute safety of water fluoridation on a long-term basis."

The Effect of Fluoride on Phagocytosis

The destruction of bacteria and other foreign agents by white cells is called phagocytosis. The process of phagocytosis is illustrated in the following diagram.

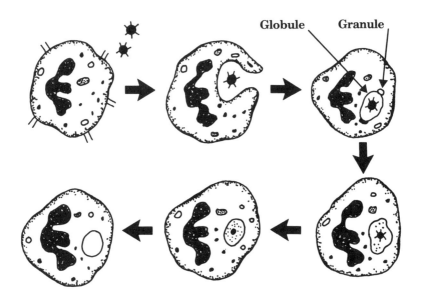

Upon reaching a foreign agent, the white blood cell encapsulates and 'swallows' it in the form of a globule. At this time, granules (within the cell) containing enzymes and co-factors necessary for the breakdown of the foreign material migrate to the globule and disappear by emptying their contents into it. A chemical called superoxide is produced by the white blood cell to aid in the ultimate destruction of the foreign agent in the globule.

Dr. Robert A. Clark from the Boston University Medical Center showed that fluoride stimulated granule formation and oxygen consumption in white blood cells when they were not challenged with a foreign agent, but inhibited these processes when the white blood cell needed them to fight off foreign agents. Similarly, Dr. W.L. Gabler and Dr. P.A. Leong at the University of Oregon Health Sciences Center found that while as little as 0.2 ppm fluoride stimulated superoxide production in resting white blood cells, the same concentration of fluoride inhibited superoxide production in white blood cells challenged with a foreign agent. John T. Curnette and co-workers from Tufts University School of Medicine found that when blood cells were exposed to fluoride *"at a concentration that stimulated vigorous O_2^- [superoxide] production by the cells, phagocytosis was virtually abolished."*

Fluoride apparently depletes the energy reserves and the ability of white blood cells to properly destroy foreign agents by the process of phagocytosis. In more recent studies, W.L. Gabler and co-workers found that at low levels of fluoride, there was a delay in the capacity of white blood cells to respond to challenges from foreign agents and that when a response occurred, it was less vigorous when fluoride was present. They pointed out: *"Since fluoride inhibits induced O_2^- [superoxide] synthesis, the practice of introducing millimolar amounts of fluoride into areas harboring potential pathogens should be questioned."* As a matter of fact, his data, as well as the data of Saito and co-workers, indicate that even micromolar amounts of fluoride, i.e. below 1 part per million, may seriously depress the ability of white blood cells to destroy pathogenic agents.

In addition, findings by these investigators and others suggest that fluoride exposure may also result in the release of superoxide from the white blood cells into the bloodstream. Increased superoxide in the bloodstream, which gives rise to tissue damage, has also been associated with an acceleration of the aging process.

A noticeable disruption in immune function has already been reported among 10- to 12-year-old children exposed to 3-5 ppm fluoride in their drinking water.

In summary, the consumption of water containing 1 part per million fluoride leads to a situation in which the ability of the body to properly dispose of foreign agents in the blood is retarded by (1) slowing down the movement of white blood cells, (2) interfering with phagocytosis, and (3) inducing the release of superoxide free radicals in resting white blood cells. This fluoride-induced interference leads to an increased and more prolonged exposure of the body to foreign materials and leads to the release of free radicals which damage the body and leads to a further acceleration of the aging process.

Fluoride Tricks and Damages the Immune System

Fluoride confuses the immune system and causes it to attack the body's own tissues. In such cases, the clinical observations of skin rashes, gastrointestinal disorders, lupus, rheumatoid arthritis, etc. are to be expected. The cumulative effect of tissue damage by these fluoride-induced autoimmune responses is what is commonly recognized as aging.

Fluoride slows down and weakens those very cells which serve as the body's defense system and thus allows foreign agents such as bacteria, viruses, and chemicals as well as the body's own obsolete, damaged or cancerous cells to wreak havoc throughout the body. Otherwise minor infections, now fighting an immune system weakened by fluoride, take longer to throw off and more serious illnesses result. Cancer cells which might otherwise be contained or destroyed end up taking the life of the victim.

This fluoride-induced weakening of the immune system explains the results of Drs. Alfred Taylor and Nell Taylor of the University of Texas who found that fluoride in the drinking water at levels of one-half to one part per million increased tumor growth rate in cancer-prone mice by 15-25%. This increased tumor growth rate can be attributed to the inability of the immune system of fluoride-treated mice to attack tumors.

WARNING: Fluoride not only causes the immune system to act like the immune system of an 'old' person, it also causes autoimmune damage to the entire body and accelerates the aging process of that body. The low levels at which fluoride exerts its deleterious effects indicates that there may be no safe level of fluoride.

Chapter 4

Breaking Down the Body's Glue

All animals, including humans, are made up of cells. The cell, the basic unit of life, can be identified under a microscope by its outer membrane and a nucleus within the membrane.

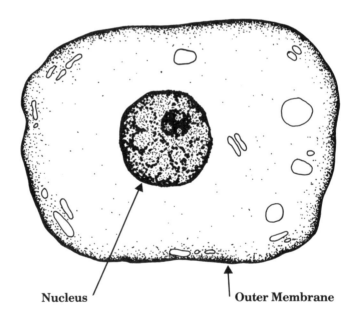

Nucleus   **Outer Membrane**

Some cells produce a protein called collagen. In this book, the term 'collagen' refers to collagen as well as other collagen-like proteins. This process occurs inside the cell. Little globules called vesicles carry the collagen from the inside of the cell to the

cell membrane where it is released to the outside of the cell.
There, the collagen thickens into fibers.

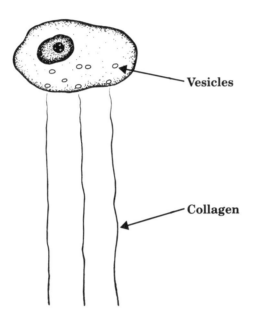

Vesicles

Collagen

The five different types of cells capable of producing and releasing collagen in this way are:
— fibroblasts, which produce collagen for the structural support of skin, tendons, ligaments and muscle;
— chondroblasts, which produce collagen for the structural support of cartilage;
— osteoblasts, which produce collagen for the structural foundation and framework upon which calcium and phosphate are deposited, giving rise to bone;
— ameloblasts, which produce collagen for the structural foundation and framework upon which calcium and phosphate are deposited, giving rise to tooth enamel;
— odontoblasts, which produce collagen for the structural foundation and framework upon which calcium and phosphate are deposited, giving rise to the inner part of the tooth. This material is called dentin.

Like other proteins, collagen is composed of amino acids linked together in a chain. However, collagen contains two additional amino acids, hydroxyproline and hydroxylysine, not found in other proteins. Thus when collagen synthesis is interfered with or when collagen breaks down, the hydroxyproline and hydroxylysine levels in the blood and urine increase.

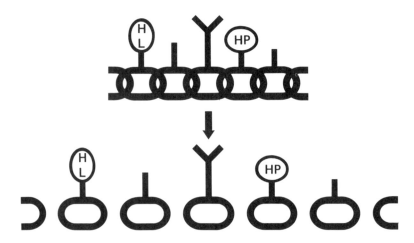

Breakdown of the collagen protein 'chain' into its amino acid 'links'. Unlike non-collagen protein the collagen protein contains hydroxyproline (HP) and hydroxylysine (HL), which are only made after the collagen chain is put together. Thus, the high levels of the 'free' hydroxyproline and hydroxylysine 'links' induced by fluoride is conclusive evidence that fluoride is accelerating the breakdown of collagen.

Researchers from Harvard University and the National Institutes of Health knew in the 1960s that fluoride disrupted collagen synthesis. It was not until 1979, however, that a new flurry of research activity in this area began.

    In 1981, Dr. Kakuya Ishida of the Kanagawa Dental University in Japan reported the results of studies in which he fed laboratory animals 1 part per million fluoride in their drinking water and analyzed the urine for hydroxyproline. He found that urinary hydroxyproline levels increased in these animals. This indicates that as little as 1 part per million fluoride interferes with collagen metabolism and leads to its breakdown.

Dr. Marian Drozdz and co-workers from the Institute of Bioanalytical and Environmental Studies in Katowice, Poland found increased hydroxyproline and hydroxylysine levels in the blood and urine as well as a decrease in skin and lung collagen levels in rats fed 1 part per million fluoride in their drinking water.

Dr. Anna Put and co-workers from the Department of Pharmacology of the Pomorska Akademy of Medicine in Szczecin, Poland also found that fluoride increased hydroxyproline levels in urine.

Drs. A.K. Susheela, Y.D. Sharma and co-workers from the All-India Institute of Medical Sciences found that fluoride exposure disrupts the synthesis of collagen and leads to the breakdown of collagen in bone, tendon, muscle, skin, cartilage, lung, kidney and trachea.

As already noted, small vesicles transport collagen from the inside of the cell to the outside of the cell. Drs. Harold Fleming and Val Greenfield of Yale University School of Medicine found a larger number of the vesicles in collagen-forming cells (ameloblasts) in animals exposed to fluoride. This work was confirmed by S. Chen and D. Eisenmann of the University of Illinois, who also found a fluoride-induced increase of these granules in ameloblasts.

It appears that fluoride disruption of collagen synthesis in cells responsible for laying down collagen leads these cells to try to compensate for their inability to put out intact collagen by producing larger quantities of imperfect collagen and/or noncollagenous protein.

In 1983, Dr. John R. Farley and co-workers from Loma Linda University showed that treatment of bone cells with less than 1 part per million fluoride increased collagen formation by 50 percent. One year later, Dr. J.R. Smid and co-workers from the Department of Oral Biology at the University of Queensland in Australia found that fluoride ingestion led to an increase of noncollagen proteins as well as collagen proteins. This is supported by the works of Drs. J.H. Bowes and M.M. Murray, Dr. Kh.A. Abishev and co-workers, and Dr. B.R. Bhussry who report a vastly higher protein content in teeth and bone damaged by fluoride. Clinical findings also show that new irregular bone growth is stimulated by fluoride.

The drawings below illustrate the effect of fluoride on collagen metabolism.

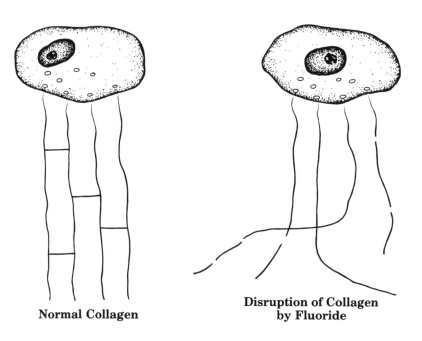

Normal Collagen   **Disruption of Collagen
                                        by Fluoride**

As mentioned above, collagen is made by many different types of cells and, under normal circumstances, is only mineralized in teeth and bones. The body obviously has some mechanism to mineralize the collagen of these tissues while leaving the collagen of other tissues, such as skin, ligaments, tendons, etc., unmineralized.

During the aging process, the body loses its ability to discriminate between which tissues should be mineralized and which tissues should not. As will be shown, consumption of fluoride results in the same loss of the body's ability to discriminate. In other words, mineralization of tissue, such as bone, which should be mineralized, is disrupted, while tendons, ligaments, muscles, and other soft tissue which should not be mineralized start to become mineralized as a result of fluoride exposure.

By interfering with collagen production, fluoride leads to the production of larger quantities of imperfect collagen and/or other types of protein and thus interferes with the body's normal regulation of collagen mineralization.

The type and array of collagen and collagen-related proteins made by the various collagen-producing cells determine whether or not the collagen framework will be mineralized. During the aging process, cumulative damage to these cells leads to the diseases attributed to 'old age' — arthritis, arteriosclerosis, brittle bones, wrinkled skin, etc. Consumption of fluoride produces the same effects and results in the same diseases.

Fluoride probably acts by interfering with the enzymes essential for setting up the proper conditions for producing intact collagen. Thus, as has already been indicated, larger amounts of imperfect or deformed collagen fibers are formed and the body's ability to regulate collagen formation and mineralization is hindered. Illustrated below is an x-ray of the forearm bone of one of a group of people with a disease attributed to the consumption of 8 to 10 mg of fluoride per day, only twice the amount of fluoride consumed by people living in fluoridated areas in the United States. The hair-like projections constitute an excellent example of collagen synthesis run wild.

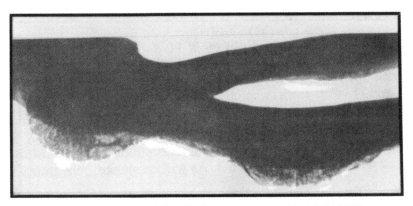

From Soriano, *Fluoride*, Volume 1, pp. 56-64 (1968)

Chapter 5

The First Visible Sign of Fluoride Poisoning: Dental Fluorosis

What happens when fluoride causes the collagen-producing cells of the tooth (ameloblasts) to go wild?

Dr. A. Bronckers and co-workers from Vrije University in Amsterdam, Holland found that in the presence of as little as 1 part per million fluoride, ameloblasts secreted an abnormal collagen matrix. Researchers from the University of North Carolina at Chapel Hill, the Dental College in Aarhus, Denmark, the Zhongshan Medical College in Canton, Peoples' Republic of China, the University of Nantes, France, and others also found that fluoride interfered with the normal function of ameloblasts in laying down collagen matrix as well as the subsequent mineralization of this enamel matrix. Depending on the degree of this interference, the tooth enamel loses its translucent appearance.

Disruption of the collagen laid down by the odontoblasts to form dentin, which makes up the structural bulk of the tooth, results in parts of the tooth fracturing off, leading to pits and even substantial parts of the tooth breaking away. Drs. W. Jarzynka and Anna Put from the Pomorska Akademy of Medicine in Szczecin, Poland and Dr. Araki from Japan showed that fluoride interferes with the mineralization of dentin.

Clinical examinations show that these dental deformities are exactly what happens after fluoride exposure.

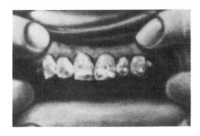 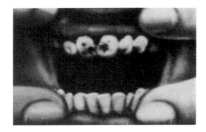

From McKay and Black, *Dental Cosmos*, **Vol. 58, pp. 447-484 (1916)**

While these types of tooth abnormalities have been known since the dawn of dentistry, it was not until 1916 that two dentists, G.V. Black and F.S. McKay, carefully listed the characteristics of these tooth deformities (which they referred to as mottled teeth) in a number of patients in the U.S. They found that in mild cases, mottling is exhibited as chalky-white areas on the tooth. In more advanced cases, teeth exhibit yellow, brown, and black stains, develop pits and crevices, and the tips break off. As other U.S. investigators became aware of this deformity, they referred to it as 'Colorado Brown Stain' or 'Texas Teeth' because mottled teeth were prevalent in those states.

Concern about this problem led three independent groups of scientists to determine, in 1931, that fluoride in the drinking water was the cause of this dental mottling. Research teams from ALCOA and the University of Arizona analyzed drinking water and found that areas that experienced this dental problem had high fluoride levels. The University of Arizona team also found that mottling could be reproduced under laboratory conditions when animals received fluoride in their drinking water. North African investigators also found that fluoride-contaminated water led to mottled teeth.

Within the next two years, similar reports concerning mottling among people from China, Argentina, Britain, Italy, and Japan were published. This led H. Trendley Dean of the United States Public Health Service to carry out a series of investigations. These investigations showed that dental mottling (now referred to as dental fluorosis) of permanent teeth of children nine years of age and over could be attributed to fluoride concentrations in the drinking water at a level slightly below 1 part per million. As fluoride levels increased above 1 part per million, so did the incidence and severity of dental fluorosis. In 1937, Dr. Dean published the following table:

DENTAL FLUOROSIS IN CHILDREN
NINE YEARS OF AGE AND OVER

City and State	Number of Children	Fluoride in Drinking Water (parts) per million	Percentage with Dental Fluorosis (Mottling)
Pueblo, CO	83	.6	2.4
Junction City, KS	115	.7	1.7
Mullins, SC	47	.9	10.6
E. Moline, IL	110	1.5	24.5
Webster City, IA	72	1.6	26.4
Monmouth, IL	38	1.7	42.1
Galesburg, IL	57	1.8	35.1
Clovis, NM	179	2.2	72.1
Colorado Spring CO	148	2.5	67.6
Plainview, TX	97	2.9	87.6
Amarillo, TX	289	3.9	90.3
Conway, SC	59	4.0	88.2
Lubbock, TX	189	4.4	97.8
Post, TX	38	5.7	100.0
Ankeny, IA	21	8.0	100.0

As can be seen from this table, there is little room for doubt that fluoride in the drinking water causes these tooth deformities.

More recently, Dr. Segretto and co-workers at the University of Texas Health Science Center Dental School in San Antonio were commissioned by the United States Environmental Protection Agency to determine the extent of fluorosis in naturally fluoridated areas. They found that children from areas with 1.0-1.4 parts per million fluoride in the water had a dental fluorosis rate 30-35% higher than children with only 0.3-0.4 part per million fluoride in their drinking water. In 1984, these investigators published their results in the ***Journal of the American Dental Association***.

Studies performed by Dennis Leverett from the University of Rochester show that 28% of children 11 to 13 years of age living in communities with water artificially fluoridated at 1 part per million had dental fluorosis. In 1986, he published the following figures showing the rates of dental fluorosis in artificially fluoridated and in nonfluoridated areas.

Percentage of Children with Dental Fluorosis in

Age	Fluoridated Communities	Nonfluoridated Communities
12	23.7%	10.1%
13	17.1%	2.3%
14	33.0%	3.5%
15	27.5%	3.0%
16	31.8%	1.7%
17	28.8%	5.3%

Dr. John Colquhoun, the Principal Dental Officer for Auckland, New Zealand also found substantially higher dental fluorosis rates among children living in fluoridated parts of Auckland (24.9%) as compared to children living in nonfluoridated parts (4.9%).

Dental fluorosis also occurs in children living in nonfluoridated areas — among those given fluoride tablets or drops or vitamin preparations containing fluoride. Dr. J.P. Brown of the University of Texas Health Science Center found that about 30% of children who were given fluoride-containing pills exhibited dental fluorosis. Dr. P.F. DePaola of the Forsyth Dental Center in Boston found that fluoride supplements were the major cause of dental fluorosis among children living in nonfluoridated areas *"particularly if ingested in tablet form prior to three years of age."* More recent research from the Royal Dental College in Aarhus, Denmark indicates that dental fluorosis can occur among children exposed to fluoride much later in life than had previously been expected, i.e., up to 7.5 to 8.5 years of age.

Cases of dental fluorosis have increased sharply in recent years and are now being reported even in areas that are not fluoridated. Food products made with fluoridated water shipped into nonfluoridated areas (such as soft drinks, reconstituted fruit juices and fruit drinks) and tea (in England and Ireland) as well as fluoride supplements are the primary reason for this increase.

Additionally, concern has been expressed about *"unaccept-able and careless methods of topical fluoride application, both in the case of high concentration [fluoride] products and home application fluorides"*. Those who are still trying to promote fluoridation blame increasing fluorosis rates on the amount of fluoride they accidentally ingest from toothpastes, gels, and mouthrinses. The amount of fluoride consumed by the average person from topical fluoride products is small compared to the amount consumed as a result of fluoridation, except in cases where children are killed in the dental chair at the dentist's office, where they are poisoned weekly in school mouth rinse programs, or where they can get into the fluoride toothpaste when their parents are not attending to them.

Dental fluorosis is more than just a cosmetic problem. It is a permanent record showing that fluoride has inter-fered with the basic life functions of the ameloblasts, the enamel forming cells, causing them to produce damaged collagen.

When calcium and phosphate are deposited on this damaged collagen foundation and framework, the distortions in the resulting tooth enamel can be seen with the naked eye. It bears repeating that this visible distortion in the tooth enamel is obvious in 20-35% of children who live in the fluoridated areas or who live in nonfluoridated areas but are given fluoride supplements.

Those who are most damaged by fluoride are undernour-ished children. According to an article published in 1952 by Drs. Maury Massler and Isaac Schour, children with lower nutri-tional status experience a higher incidence of dental fluorosis after drinking water containing fluoride levels of about 1 part per million. As the following table shows, they found that dental

fluorosis occurs in 60% of the undernourished children of
Quarto, Italy exposed to 1.3 parts per million fluoride in their
drinking water.

DENTAL FLUOROSIS IN QUARTO, ITALY AND JOLIET, ILLINOIS

	Quarto, Italy	**Joliet, IL**
Fluoride content of water supply (in part per million)	1.3	1.3
Percentage of children with mottling	60.0	25.3
Index of dental fluorosis	1.20	0.46
Nutritional status of population	Very poor	Good

Comparing the rates of dental fluorosis in Quarto, Italy and
Joliet, Illinois, Drs. Massler and Schour conclude: *"The higher
index of mottling in Italy may be explained on the basis of difference in nutritional status. It appears that as the nutritional
status is lowered, the cells (ameloblasts) which are responsible for
the formation and calcification of the enamel become more
susceptible to the deleterious action of fluorine."*

Ironically, even though the U.S. National Institute of Dental
Research has found that as little as 0.4-0.8 parts per million
fluoride in the drinking water causes mottled teeth, 1 part per
million fluoride has actually been added to public water supplies
in the United States, in an attempt to improve dental health.
Evidence, however, suggests that older life-long residents of
naturally fluoridated areas experience a greater number of
missing teeth than in nonfluoridated areas. This was experienced by the villagers of Turkey and India as previously discussed in Chapter 1. More extensive studies have shown the
same result in areas such as Hartlepoole, England, where the
drinking water has a natural fluoride content of 2 parts per
million.

As devastating as the visible effects of dental fluorosis might appear, these damaged teeth are merely a reflection of the metabolic disturbances of soft tissue cells referred to as amelo-blasts and odontoblasts. These teeth then become a permanent record that tooth-forming cells were poisoned during tooth development. There is no question that disruption of collagen, while not always visible, occurs in the teeth of all children drinking fluoridated water or taking fluoride supplements. Furthermore, many soft tissue cells do not produce collagen. Therefore the damage done to these cells will not be reflected in visibly detectable deformities but rather in more insidious biochemical disturbances which will be discussed later. In the next two chapters the symptoms as well as the expected symp-toms that result from fluoride poisoning of other collagen-producing cells will be presented.

WARNING: While the visible symptoms of dental fluorosis occur in only 20-35% of those consuming fluori-dated drinking water or fluoride supplements during childhood, premature loss of teeth can still be expected to occur even in those who do not exhibit dental fluorosis due to damage caused during tooth develop-ment.

Chapter 6

Aging the Bone: The Degenerative Effects of Skeletal Fluorosis

Now let's look at the bone. Unlike the ameloblasts and odonto-blasts of teeth whose regenerative activity stops after tooth development, osteoblasts continue to actively lay down collagen, and new bone formation continues to take place.

If a tooth breaks or fractures, you're out of luck. The damage cannot be repaired. However, if a bone breaks or fractures, osteoblasts lay down collagen to produce a framework for new bone formation to repair the damage.

Bone also has the ability to rejuvenate itself. As older bone is removed by bone scavenger cells called osteoclasts, osteoblasts lay down collagen to produce a framework for new bone formation to renew the skeletal structure.

Thus, damage to collagen production in bone can interfere with the normal processes of bone rejuvenation and repair throughout life.

Cartilage

The balls and sockets of bones are lined with a smooth, tough elastic substance called cartilage. Maintaining the integrity of cartilage depends largely upon the ability of cells called chondroblasts to lay down noncalcified collagen which is the major structural component of cartilage.

The Effect of Fluoride on Bone and Cartilage

Fluoride has been shown to interfere with collagen formation in osteoblasts and chondroblasts. Since this increased production of imperfect collagen or collagen-like protein results in mineralization of tissues which should not be mineralized, and vice versa, one would expect a calcification of ligaments, cartilage, and tendons as well as the formation of poorly and overly mineralized bone. This is exactly what happens after exposure to fluoride.

In discussing their examination of tissues from patients exposed to fluoride, Drs. A. Singh and S.S. Jolly, internationally recognized experts on the clinical effects of fluoride on bone, point out that:

— The most noticeable changes are detected in the spine, with calcification of various spinal ligaments, resulting in pronounced bony outgrowths. The other bones show numerous spiky outgrowths especially in tendons (collagen-rich fibrous tissues which attach muscles to bone) and ligaments (collagen-rich fibrous tissues which hold bones together). Under careful inspection, the bony outgrowths are found to consist of coarse, woven fibers which are largely uncalcified.

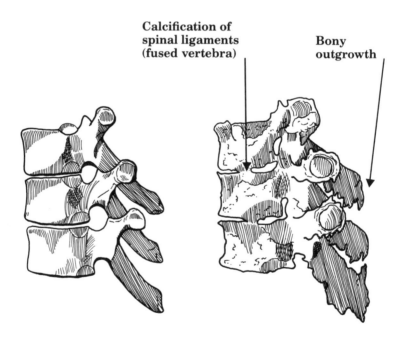

Calcification of spinal ligaments (fused vertebra)

Bony outgrowth

Normal Spinal Vertebrae

Fluoride-induced Damage to Spinal Vertebrae

— Irregular bone is also laid down in joint sockets. . .

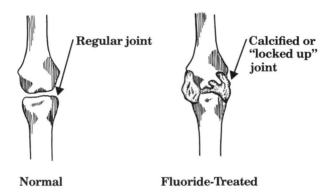

Normal   Fluoride-Treated

and interosseous membranes (membranes between bones in arms and legs).

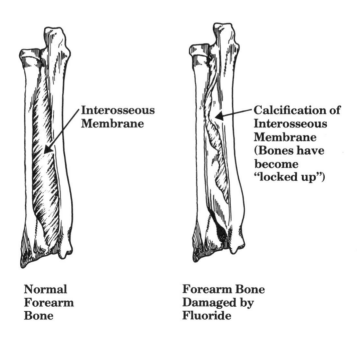

Normal   Forearm Bone
Forearm   Damaged by
Bone   Fluoride

— In more advanced cases of fluoride exposure, bones become held together by masses of new bony tissue laid down in the joint socket, ligaments, and tendons. This results in the locking up of joints and the permanent inability of victims to move or flex their joints. Vertebrae become fused at many places. This results in the characteristic 'hunch back' syndrome of skeletal fluorosis.

— There is a low degree of mineralization of the bone itself, which is partly due to a wide seam of uncalcified osteoid (collagen).

In 1973, Dr. Jolly and co-workers presented radiological evidence that skeletal fluorosis which results in these bone deformities occurs in parts of India where the drinking water contains as little as 0.7 parts per million fluoride and that the occurrence and severity increases with increasing levels of fluoride in the drinking water.

RADIOLOGICAL EVIDENCE OF SKELETAL
FLUOROSIS IN MALES 21 YEARS
OF AGE AND OLDER

Village	Water Fluoride (ppm)	Percentage
Mandi Baretta	.7	2.8
Kooriwara	2.3	40.0
Gurnay Kalan	2.4	19.6
Ganza Dhanaula	4.2	26.3
Bajakhana	5.1	46.9
Rajia	5.2	52.2
Village Baretta	5.5	29.6
Rorki	7.0	52.5
Saideke	8.2	52.6
Khara	9.4	80.1

Once thought to be a disease confined to India, skeletal fluorosis is being found world-wide as diagnostic techniques improve and an awareness of its existence increases. A French study showed that out of 29 people diagnosed with skeletal fluorosis, 14 drank bottled water (St. Yorre-Royale) containing 8.5 ppm fluoride, four obtained fluoride through their drinking water, two received fluoride in medications, and one was exposed to fluoride at work. Other cases of skeletal fluorosis include a 54-year-old woman from a region in the United States where the levels of fluoride in the drinking water ranged from 4 to 8 ppm who was diagnosed as having skeletal fluorosis and a middle-aged male from Libya living in an area containing 1-2 ppm fluoride. The latter individual also was noted to have consumed copious amounts of tea since childhood (see Chapter 12).

In 1985, Dr. I. Arnala and co-workers of Kuopio University in Finland reported that: *"The upper limit for fluoride concentration in drinking water that does not increase the amount of mineralized bone is roughly 1.5 parts per million. . . . We should however, recognize that it is difficult to give a strict value for a safe concentration in drinking water because individual susceptibility to fluoride varies."*

In addition to fluoride-induced bone abnormalities, one could expect that fluoride-induced irregularities of the joint cartilage (which is normally smooth) would result in the irritation and inflammation commonly referred to as arthritis. One could also expect fluoride to cause an increase in the incidence of fractures and a decrease in the body's ability to heal bone breaks and bone fractures.

Clinical observations show that this is exactly what happens.

Arthritic Changes

Drs. Singh and Jolly point out that early symptoms of fluoride-induced damage to bones and cartilage start with *"vague pains noted most frequently in the small joints of the spine. These cases are frequent in the endemic [local] areas and may be misdiagnosed as rheumatoid or osteoarthritis.*

"In later stages, there is an obvious stiffness of the spine with limitation of movements, and still later, the development of kyphosis [hunch back].

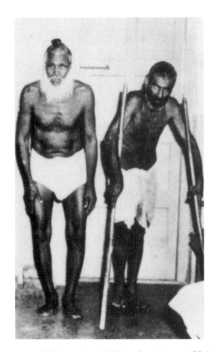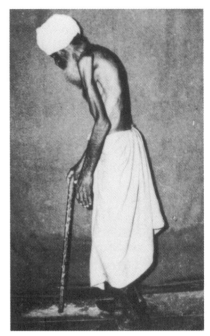

"There is difficulty in walking, due partly to stiffness and limitation of the movements of various joints. . .

"Some patients complain of dyspnea [difficulty in breathing] on exertion because of the rigidity of the thoracic cage."

In the United States, Dr. George Waldbott also diagnosed some of the early symptoms listed above, including arthritis and joint pains, as being due to the consumption of water fluoridated at 1 part per million. He was able to bring about a reversal in these symptoms by eliminating fluoridated water from his patients' diets. However, if left unattended, this degeneration will lead to the advanced stages of arthritis and 'old age'.

Similar arthritic symptoms have been reported among people exposed to air-borne fluoride emitted by fluoride-polluting industries in Switzerland, Germany, Britain, United States, Canada , and North Africa. Dr. Yiamouyiannis was contacted by a British broadcasting company concerning a problem they had found in a brick manufacturing area about 50 miles outside of London where they reported that over 90% of the population was suffering from arthritis induced by air-borne fluoride.

Dr. Waldbott noted the possibility of the age-accelerating effects of fluoride with respect to arthritis and stated:

"Among the elderly, arthritis of the spine is an especially common ailment that is customarily attributed to 'aging'. Since fluoride retention in bones increases as a person grows older, how can we disregard the possibility that this 'old age' disease might be linked with fluoride intake? For example. . .[others have] described in detail X-ray changes encountered in skeletal fluorosis in North Africa that are in every respect identical to those present in the arthritic spine of the elderly."

Breaks and Fractures

In 1978, Dr. J.A. Albright and co-workers from Yale University reported at the Annual Meeting of the Orthopedics Research Society that as little as 1 part per million fluoride decreases bone strength and elasticity.

In 1983, Dr. B. Uslu from Anadelu University School of Medicine in Eskisehir, Turkey reported that addition of fluoride to the drinking water of rats with fractured bones resulted in defective healing of the fracture due to disruption of collagen synthesis.

In 1990, Dr. Steven Jacobsen and co-workers found a link between the rate of hip fracture among U.S. women 65 years of age and over and the degree of fluoridation in their county of residence. This study examined the records of 541,985 cases of osteoporosis and was published in the ***Journal of the American Medical Association***. Another study done in Britain reported similar results for men and women 45 years of age and over. In this study, it was found that increasing the concentration of fluoride in the water from 0 to 1 ppm would increase the hip fracture rate by about 40%. A Utah study, also published in the ***Journal of the American Medical Association***, reported a fluoridation-linked 41% increase in hip fracture rate among men 65 years of age and older and a 27% increase in hip fracture rate among women 65 years of age.

At higher concentrations of fluoride in the drinking water, these effects increase. Women living in a community with 4 ppm fluoride in their drinking water were found to have a significantly lower radial bone mass, an increased rate of radial bone mass loss (in premenopausal women), and significantly more fractures (among postmenopausal women) than women living in a community with 1 ppm fluoride in their drinking water.

Drs. L. Zong-Chen and Wu En-Huei reported that in persons drinking water containing 5 ppm fluoride, osteoporosis was one of the first signs of bone damage, followed by ossification of interosseus membranes, degeneration of joints, osteomalacia, bone demineralization and other bone irregularities.

It is difficult to believe that anyone would ever think of treating osteoporosis (a disease in which the bones lose calcium) with fluoride, a substance which leads to decalcification of bone, but they have — and at doses exceeding those mentioned above.

Commenting on the results of this insane treatment in 1978, the *Journal of the American Medical Association* published an editorial pointing out that *"in several short-term studies, fluoride has been administered for treatment of involutional osteoporosis, alone or with supplemental calcium, vitamin D or both. No studies have demonstrated alleviation of fracture[s]. . . However, studies have shown an increased incidence of . . . fractures. When high doses of fluorides have been given to animals receiving a diet that was otherwise unchanged, most studies have shown no change or a decrease in the strength of the bone."* They also pointed out that administration of fluoride resulted in nonmineralized seams in bones, resulting in the disease called osteomalacia.

In 1980, Dr. J.C. Robin and co-workers from the Roswell Park Memorial Institute confirmed the foolishness of using fluoride for the treatment of osteoporosis. In the *Journal of Medicine*, they wrote, *"fluoride had no preventative effect. In some experiments there was even a deleterious effect of fluoride."* They found fluoride accelerated the process of osteoporosis, leading to a loss of calcium from the bone.

In 1986, additional studies were published implying and/or showing that fluoride treatment was causing osteoporosis and bone fractures. M. A. Dumbacher and co-workers from the University of Zurich found a substantial increase in the bone fracture rate in osteoporosis patients treated with fluoride compared to those who were not. At a meeting in Nice, France, Dr. Lawrence Riggs of the Mayo Clinic declined to respond to the press regarding a report he delivered indicating that fluoride might accelerate the loss of bone mass in the hips and long bones. However, four years later, he published an article in the *New England Journal of Medicine* concluding that fluoride treatment of osteoporosis *"increases skeletal fragility"*. His results showed that the bone fracture rate in osteoporosis patients treated with fluoride was about 40% higher than in patients not treated with fluoride. He reported that fluoride treatment was linked to an increase in nonvertebral fractures 3 times as high as that of nontreated patients.

In the meantime, similar results poured in from many other clinics and hospitals. C. M. Schnitzler and co-workers reported an increase in bone fragility during fluoride therapy for osteoporosis. This led to increases in stress fractures and spinal fractures. The nonvertebral fracture rate of fluoride-treated patients was three times that of untreated patients.

L. R. Hedlund and J. C. Gallagher examined hip fracture rates in 22 untreated patients, 21 patients treated without fluoride, and 35 patients treated with fluoride. After two years, 6 hip fractures were observed — and all of them occurred in the fluoride-treated group.

And that's not all. Fluoride treatment of osteoporosis has other serious side-effects, all of which are predictable. It has been shown to cause pain and swelling of joints, gastric pain, vomiting, gastrointestinal bleeding, anemia, bone spurs, pain in the lower extremities, arthritis, periostitis, and possible cancerous transformations in white blood cells.

High fluoride doses are also obtained when fluoridated tap water is used in artificial kidney machines. In 1973, a report from the National Institute of Arthritis and Metabolic Diseases found 50 to 100% increases in the incidence of a disease called osteitis fibrosa among patients whose artificial kidney machines were run on fluoridated water. Osteitis fibrosa is a disease characterized by fibrous degeneration of the bone; it results in bone deformities and sometimes in fracture.

Bony Outgrowths

Even the bony outgrowths attributed to the increased synthesis of imperfect collagen or collagen-like proteins can give rise to deformities and discomfort. Illustrated below is an example of what can result from consuming wine contaminated with small amounts of fluoride.

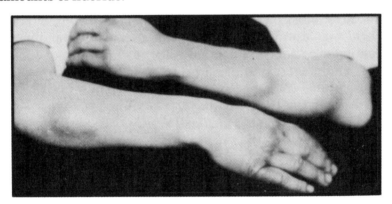

Premature Aging of the Bone

Drs. A.F. Aksyuk and G.V. Bulychev from the Erisman Research Institute in Moscow found that the consumption of 1.6 parts per million fluoride in the drinking water led to premature calcification and aging of the bones of the majority of 15- to 16-year-old girls that they had examined. They also noticed that these girls had a tendency to calcify the interosseous membranes (membranes between bones in arms and legs). This results in irregular bone formation (see page 49).

According a *New York Times* article dated October 28, 1992,

Sports Injuries to the Young Are Up Sharply, Doctors Say

"Adults recall childhood as an endless blur of running and jumping, full of little cuts and bruises, but blissfully free of those nagging injuries that follow exercise later in life — tendinitis, bursitis and stress fractures.

"Now, however, orthopedists and pediatricians say these injuries are cropping up with alarming frequency in children: from stress fractures of the lower spine in young gymnasts to shoulder tendinitis in swimmers to shin splints in aspiring marathoners.

"'People are suddenly recognizing that it's a problem', said Dr. Carl L. Stanitski, chief of orthopedic surgery at the Children's Hospital of Michigan in Detroit. 'We are seeing more and more stress fractures in children and more and more injuries cause by repetitive use.'".

Pathological Effects

Fluoride affects bones and teeth by interfering with the production of collagen. A common belief that damage caused by fluoride results from higher fluoride levels in the mineral parts of these tissues is no longer acceptable and cannot explain the disruptive effects of fluoride for the following reasons:

— It has never been shown that the fluoride content is any higher in damaged teeth or bone than in undamaged teeth or bone, in either the same person or in different persons exposed to the same concentrations of fluoride in the environment.

— Some bones and teeth with no obvious irregularities have been shown to contain more fluoride than the amount found in fluoride-damaged bones and teeth.

Thus, like lead and strontium-90, even though fluoride accumulates primarily in the mineralized part of bone, it does not exhibit its toxic effect due merely to its presence there. Fluoride damage is caused by its biochemical effects on living cells which give rise to bone and tooth formation, as well as other cells (see the following chapter).

WARNING: While arthritis and other clinical manifestations of bone disease do not occur in everyone drinking fluoridated water, processes leading to the premature development of arthritis, osteoporosis, and bone fragility can be expected to occur in all people who drink fluoridated water or who, in any other way, increase their fluoride intake.

Chapter 7

Premature Aging: Skin, Arteries, Other Tissues

In addition to the bones, teeth, and cartilage, a number of soft tissues contain cells which synthesize collagen. These cells are called fibroblasts. Fibroblasts produce the collagen which becomes the major structural component of skin, arteries, muscles, tendons, and ligaments. In contrast to the collagen of bones and teeth, the collagen synthesized by fibroblasts, under normal circumstances, remains uncalcified.

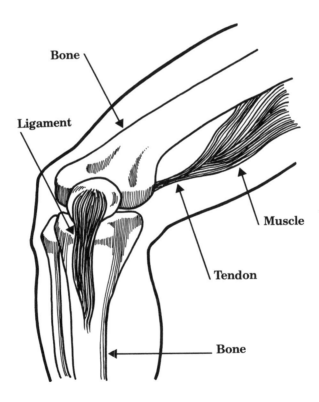

Muscle cells are surrounded by collagen fibers which provide support and prevent the muscle from ripping. Near the ends of muscle tissues, the number of muscle cells decreases, resulting in more and more collagen until a point is reached where there are no more muscle cells and only collagen is left (along with a few fibroblasts). This is called the tendon. As the tendon approaches the bone, the tendon collagen merges with bone collagen, thereby forming a bridge of collagen connecting the muscle to the bone. Similarly, ligaments form a 'collagen bridge' from one bone to another.

Ligaments also form a network of fibers throughout the abdominal cavity which holds other tissues and organs, such as the liver, kidney, and uterus, in place.

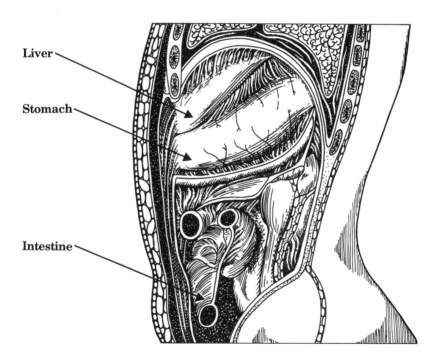

An illustration of the abdominal cavity. All the fibrous tissues in this diagram are ligaments. These ligaments (collagen) attach the various organs to the abdominal wall which itself is lined with ligamentous material.

As pointed out earlier, disruption of collagen metabolism leads to the calcification of tissue which should not be calcified and a reduction of calcification in tissue which should be calcified.

After careful examination of the tissues of people exposed to fluoride, Drs. Singh and Jolly found calcified ligaments, tendons, and muscles. They even noticed a calcification of thyroid cartilage in some cases.

Hardening of the Arteries

In a number of areas where people consume water containing 3 parts per million fluoride or more, calcification of the arteries has been clinically correlated with the fluoride-induced bone disorders described in Chapter 6. The indication again is that fibroblasts in the arterial cell walls are producing larger amounts of an imperfect collagen or collagen-like protein, resulting in hardening of the arteries or arteriosclerosis, the leading cause of death in the United States.

During aging, hardening of the arteries is probably due to disruption of collagen production, according to Dr. John Negalesko, director of the first year medical program at the Ohio State University Medical School and an expert in the field. Thus, fluoride, by disrupting the production of collagen and by stimulating the calcification of arteries, can speed up another phase of the aging process.

Skin

Since collagen is the primary structural material of skin, damage to skin collagen can be expected to lead to the prematurely wrinkled skin of the people of Kizilcaoern, referred to in Chapter 1. The wrinkling itself may be due either to a breakdown in collagen structure or to a slight calcification of the skin collagen or both.

Calcification of skin collagen is a well-known phenomenon. It is called scleroderma. People experiencing scleroderma also experience hardening or calcification of the arteries (arteriosclerosis), arthritis, hardening of the ligamentous material supporting the internal organs, and osteoporosis — the same symptoms that result from fluoride exposure. In fact, scleroderma has been found in about 50% of the workers employed in an aluminum plant as a result of exposure to hydrogen fluoride as well as other fluorides.

Another characteristic of scleroderma is the production of excessive amounts of collagen in skin tissue, in heart muscle, in arteries, in lung and in kidney. These are the same pathological conditions that are predictable effects of fluoride.

Excessive production of collagen in scleroderma results in the loss of muscle cells as well as other soft tissues cells leading to loss of muscular activity and/or neuromuscular incoordination. And in fact Dr. George Waldbott, after examining 400 cases of pathological reactions attributable to fluoride exposure, has reported muscular weakness and lack of coordination as a result.

Before the onset of these fluoride-induced diseases becomes clinically detectable, adverse health effects will occur. The peak performance of athletes will be hindered by subclinical muscular weakness as well as torn ligaments and tendons. Arteriosclerosis, by restricting blood flow to the brain, will lead to premature senility. Other diseases such as muscular dystrophy, rheumatoid arthritis, and lupus may also be set off by fluoride's disruptive effect on collagen in soft tissues.

Chapter 8

Genetic Damage

As pointed out in Chapter 4, all animals, including humans, are made up of cells. Each cell contains a nucleus, which is separated from the remainder of the cell by a nuclear membrane. Within the nucleus exist chromosomes, which contain DNA and protein. DNA is the body's master blueprint material. It is the genetic material that determines how the body is built. DNA specifies traits such as height, hair texture and color, number of fingers on each hand, blood type, and by means of its control of protein and enzyme synthesis, the susceptibility of the individual to various diseases.

Nucleus   Chromosomes

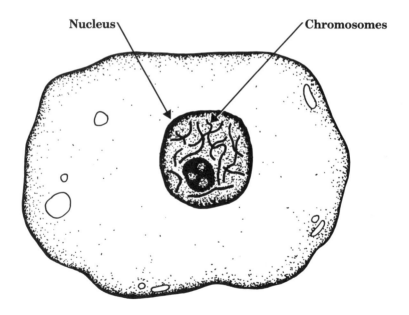

Since maintaining the integrity of this master blueprint is so vital, the cell makes a 'photocopy' of the DNA called RNA, so that the risk of damaging the DNA is minimized. This photocopy blueprint is taken to 'construction sites' in the cell. These construction sites are called ribosomes. On these ribosomes, the RNA blueprint is used to direct the manufacture of proteins and enzymes, which, in turn, directly determine the structure, traits, and limiting capabilities of the body.

To further insure the integrity of DNA, the cell provides a group of enzymes called the DNA repair enzyme system which repairs DNA when damage is done to it. As people age, their DNA repair enzyme systems slow down. This results in DNA damage which goes unrepaired and leads to cell damage or death. Damaged or dead cells may then put out products which in turn damage other cells, leading eventually to massive cell death and the degenerative loss of various tissues and organs in a snowballing cycle of aging -> damage -> aging . . .

Serious consequences can also arise if the unrepaired DNA damage occurs in a cell which gives rise to a sperm or egg cell. In these cases, DNA damage in the defective egg or sperm cell will be replicated in every cell of the offspring's body and will lead to a birth defect. If the child with this birth defect survives to maturity and reproduces, this genetic deformity will be passed on from generation to generation. A decline in DNA repair activity with 'age' is one of the reasons why the incidence of birth defects increases as maternal age increases.

Unrepaired damage of a segment of the DNA responsible for control of cell growth (brought about by a deficient DNA repair enzyme system) can lead to uncontrolled cell growth or tumors. Many tumors stop growing when they are contained by the cells around them. However, in some cases, tumor cells may release an enzyme, which digests the surrounding cells. The result is an invasive or malignant tumor — more commonly referred to as cancer.

An excellent example of a defective DNA repair enzyme system leading to cancer is provided by victims of a disease called xeroderma pigmentosum. These people suffer from an inherited deficiency of DNA repair enzyme activity and are known to succumb to cancer early in life as a result.

A decline in DNA repair activity with 'age' is one of the primary reasons why the incidence of cancer among older people is so much higher than the cancer incidence among younger people. The defective DNA repair enzyme in patients with xeroderma pigmentosum accelerates the aging process to the extent that xeroderma pigmentosum patients in their 20s have the same cancer risk as 'normal' people in their 80s.

Dr. Wolfgang Klein and co-workers at the Seibersdorf Research Center in Austria reported that 1 part per million fluoride inhibits DNA repair enzyme activity by 50%. Since fluoride inhibits DNA repair enzyme activity, fluoride should also be expected to lead to an increase in genetic or chromosome damage.

This has indeed been found to occur in numerous studies showing that fluoride in water, even at the concentration of 1 part per million, can cause chromosome damage.

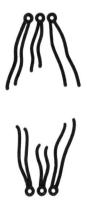

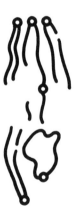

Normal Chromosomes   **Damaged Chromosomes**

The following table outlines the results of laboratory studies
regarding the effect of fluoride on genetic damage in mammals.

Year	Institution	Animal	Findings
1973	Russian Research Institute of Industrial Health and Occupational Diseases	rat	fluoride causes genetic damage
1974	Columbia University College of Physicians and Surgeons (USA)	mouse/ sheep/cow	fluoride causes genetic damage
1978	Pomeranian Medical Academy (Poland)	human blood cells	fluoride causes genetic damage
1979	National Institute of Dental Research (USA)	mouse	fluoride does not* cause genetic damage
1981	Institute of Botany, Baku (USSR)	rat (3 studies)	fluoride causes genetic damage
1982	University of Missouri, Kansas City (USA)	mouse	fluoride causes genetic damage
1983	Kunming Institute of Zoology (Peop. Rep. China)	deer	fluoride causes genetic damage
1983	Kunming Institute of Zoology (Peop. Rep. China)	human blood cells	fluoride causes genetic damage
1984	Nippon Dental University, Tokyo (Japan)	hamster embryo cell	fluoride causes genetic damage
1984	Nippon Dental University, Tokyo (Japan)	human cell culture	fluoride causes genetic damage

1984	Tokyo Medical and Dental University (Japan)	human blood cells	fluoride causes genetic damage
1985	Medical Research Council, Edinburgh (UK)	human blood cells	fluoride causes genetic damage
1986	University of Sussex (UK)	mouse lymphoma cells	fluoride causes genetic damage
1987	Paterson Institute for Cancer Research (UK)	human cell culture	fluoride causes genetic damage
1987	National Institute of Environmental Health Sciences (USA)	mouse lymphoma cells	fluoride causes genetic damage
1987	ICI Pharmaceuticals (UK)	human blood cells	fluoride causes genetic damage
1987	Institute of Pitaniia (USSR)	rat bone marrow cells	fluoride causes genetic damage
1989	Proctor and Gamble (USA)	hamster ovary cells	fluoride causes genetic damage
1989	Nippon Dental University, Tokyo (Japan)	human cell culture	fluoride causes genetic damage

---

*A prepublication copy of this paper was submitted as an exhibit in a court case in Pittsburgh (USA). During trial, it was brought out that the results showed that increasing the fluoride content of drinking water increased genetic damage in mouse testes cells. Before the paper was published these figures were altered so as to destroy the original figures showing a relation between fluoride and genetic damage (see Chapter 16).

Among the most relevant of these studies are those of Dr. Aly Mohamed, a geneticist at the University of Missouri. They show that one part per million fluoride in the drinking water of mice causes chromosomal damage. These studies also show that as the fluoride content of the water increases, the degree of chromosomal damage increases in both testes and bone marrow. The results are presented in the following table:

CHROMOSOME DAMAGE CAUSED BY FLUORIDE

Fluoride (ppm)	Percent of Cells with Chromosomal Damage			
	Bone Marrow		Testes	
	3 weeks	6 weeks	3 weeks	6 weeks
0	18.4	19.3	16.0	15.8
1	25.7	32.1	21.4	21.1
5	29.9	41.3	23.2	22.8
10	35.5	46.0	30.5	29.7
50	44.6	47.1	34.3	41.3
100	47.5	47.9	40.3	48.2
200	45.6	49.2	42.5	50.3

Chromosomes (and thus any chromosomal abnormalities that may occur) are only visible while the cell is dividing. Therefore, Dr. Mohamed studied bone marrow and testes cells because they divide rapidly.

Since the testes cells give rise to sperm cells which are passed on to future generations, genetic damage to these testes cells can lead to birth defects and other metabolic disorders which can be passed on from generation to generation.

Studies by Procter and Gamble showed that fluoride at levels of less than 1ppm caused genetic damage in Chinese hamster ovary cells, as can be seen from the following table, which summarizes the statistically significant data from a paper they published in *Mutation Research* in 1989.

CHROMOSOME DAMAGE CAUSED BY FLUORIDE

Fluoride (ppm)	Percent of Cells with Chromosomal Damage
0	2
.5	6
11	8
23	16
34	29
45	32

Early studies regarding the ability of fluoride to cause chromo-somal damage were done on plants and insects and as a result drew little attention. However, since the basic structure, func-tion, and repair of chromosomes is similar in plants, insects, and animals, substances like fluoride which cause genetic damage in plants and insects, will most likely cause genetic damage in animals — including man.

The following table outlines the results of laboratory studies regarding the effect of fluoride on genetic damage in plants and insects.

Year	Institution	Plant or Insect Used	Findings
1966	Texas A& M University (USA)	Onion	fluoride causes genetic damage
1966	Texas A & M University (USA)	Tomato	fluoride causes genetic damage
1968	University of Missouri Kansas City (USA)	Tomato	fluoride causes genetic damage
1970	University of Missouri Kansas City (USA)	Maize	fluoride causes genetic damage
1970	University of Missouri Kansas City (USA)	Fruit Fly	fluoride causes genetic damage

1971	Texas A&M University (USA)	Fruit Fly	fluoride causes genetic damage
1973	Texas A&M University (USA)	Fruit Fly	fluoride causes genetic damage
1973	Central Laboratory for Mutagen Testing (W. Germany)	Fruit Fly	fluoride causes genetic damage
1973	Texas A&M University (USA)	Barley (2)	fluoride causes genetic damage
1982	Institute of Botany Baku (USSR)	Onion	fluoride causes genetic damage
1983:	Institute of Botany Baku (USSR)	Onion	fluoride causes genetic damage

Drs. R.N. Mukherjee and F.H. Sobels from the University of Leiden in Holland found that fluoride increased the frequency of genetic damage in sperm cells of laboratory animals exposed to X-rays. It is evident from their studies that fluoride inhibited the repair of DNA damaged by X-rays. The authors concluded: *"sodium fluoride resulted in a consistent and highly significant increase of the mutation [i.e. genetic damage] frequency. This effect is thought to result from interference with a repair process."*

In agreement with Drs. Mukherjee and Sobels were Dr. S.I. Voroshilin and co-workers from the Russian Research Institute of Industrial Health and Occupational Diseases. From their studies they concluded: *"It would seem to us that fluoride could cause some kind of disturbance in the enzymes that are related to the mechanisms of DNA repair and synthesis."*

Dr. Danuta Jachimczak and co-workers from the Pomeranian Medical Academy in Poland reported that as little as 0.6 part per million fluoride produces chromosomal damage in human white blood cells. This study has received support from two other studies by Dr. R. Lin and co-workers from the Kunming Institute of Zoology and Dr. E.J. Thomson and co-workers from the Medical Research Council in Edinburgh, Scotland, who showed a 2-fold to 15-fold increase in chromosomal aberration rates at levels of 1.5 to 60 parts per million fluoride. The Thomson study suffers from the fact that the investigators administered another mutagenic substance to all the cells tested to measure other indexes of chromosomal activity.

Dr. Stephen Greenberg from the Chicago Medical School observed a disturbance of the DNA in white blood cells of animals treated with 5-10 ppm fluoride and observed other changes which he maintained were characteristic of cancer cells.

It is quite clear that fluoride causes genetic damage. The mechanism of action of fluoride cannot be exactly pinpointed because fluoride interferes with a number of physiological processes. Most evidence indicates that fluoride acts on the DNA repair enzyme system. This does not rule out the possibility that fluoride also interferes with DNA synthesis or that it may even act directly on the DNA itself. DNA is composed of two molecular strands held together by hydrogen bonds and fluoride is capable of disrupting these bonds. Such disruption would be expected to result in genetic damage directly and/or interference with DNA synthesis and DNA repair. Fluoride-induced genetic damage may also result from the general metabolic imbalance caused by fluoride selectively inhibiting certain enzymes.

Birth Defects

In 1981, Dr. A. Iarez and co-workers from the Department of Toxicology from Central University of Venezuela in Caracas reported that fluoride added to the drinking water of female rats produced birth defects in their offspring. Just one year later Drs. Rhuitao Zhang and Shunguang Zhang of the Changjian Institute of Marine Products found that fluoride caused birth defects in fish.

In 1992, Dr. L. Du from the Department of Pathology, Guiyang Medical College in China found cellular abnormalities in brain tissue indicating that chronic fluorosis in the course of intrauterine fetal life may produce certain harmful effects on the developing brain of the fetus.

According to the June 16, 1976 issue of the ***San Diego Union***, an experiment showed that 10% of the litters of female mice drinking tap water from Durham, North Carolina (fluoridated in 1962) contained at least one malformed baby. No birth defects were observed in mice drinking purified water. While this study in itself does not prove that fluoride was the cause, the effects of fluoride mentioned above certainly make it a prime suspect.

Chapter 9

Cancer

"Everything causes cancer? Perhaps. Conceivably even a single electron at the other side of the universe. The real question is, how likely is any one particular cause? In point of fact, fluoride causes more human cancer death, and causes it faster, than any other chemical."

> Dean Burk
> Chief Chemist Emeritus
> U.S. National Cancer Institute

Substances like fluoride which cause genetic damage are called mutagenic substances, and it is a well-accepted fact that substances which are mutagenic also tend to be carcinogenic, or cancer-producing. In fact, this is exactly what has been found with regard to fluoride.

In 1984, Dr. Takeki Tsutsui and co-workers of the Nippon Dental College in Japan showed that fluoride not only caused genetic damage but was also capable of transforming normal cells into cancer cells. The levels of fluoride used in this study were the same levels of fluoride that the U.S. National Cancer Institute suggested should be used to determine whether or not fluoridation of public water supplies causes cancer.

These researchers found that cells treated with 34 and 45 parts per million fluoride produced cancer (fibrosarcoma) when injected under the skin of otherwise healthy adult hamsters. In contrast they found that cells that were not treated with fluoride did not produce cancer.

In 1988, researchers from the Argonne National Laboratories and others confirmed the cancer-causing ability of fluoride found by Tsutsui and coworkers. The researchers from Argonne National Laboratories also found that fluoride promotes and enhances the carcinogenicity of other cancer-causing chemicals.

These results confirm the earlier U.S. National Cancer Institute-sponsored studies done by Drs. Irwin Herskowitz and Isabel Norton. In 1963, these St. Louis University scientists showed that low levels of fluoride increased the incidence of melanotic tumors in fruit flies by 12% to 100% (see the following figure).

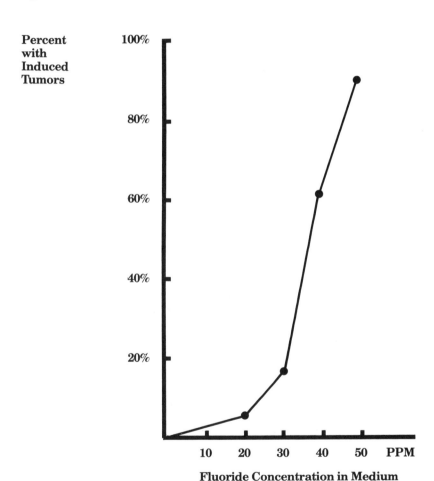

Within a matter of days, fluoride induced tumors in these experimental animals (from Herskowitz and Norton)

Similar types of transformations of normal cells to potentially cancerous cells have been observed in humans. Dr. Paul H. Duffey and co-workers from the Tucson Medical Center found that certain white blood cells were transformed into cells which appeared to be cancerous during the treatment of an osteoporosis patient with fluoride. After discontinuance of the fluoride treatments, the cancer-like cells disappeared.

Based on the studies of Herskowitz and Norton and Duffey, as well as studies by Drs. Taylor and Taylor from the University of Texas at Austin which found that one part per million fluoride in the drinking water increased tumor growth rate in mice by 25%, Dr. Dean Burk, former chief chemist of the National Cancer Institute, and Dr. John Yiamouyiannis began a series of studies to determine whether they could observe an increase in cancer death rates among human populations after fluoridation of their water supplies.

They compared the cancer death rate of the ten largest fluoridated cities with the cancer death rate of the ten largest nonfluoridated cities that had comparable cancer death rates from 1940 to 1950, a period of time during which neither group of cities was fluoridated.

Fluoridated Cities	Nonfluoridated Cities
Chicago	Los Angeles
Philadelphia	Boston
Baltimore	New Orleans
Cleveland	Seattle
Washington	Cincinnati
Milwaukee	Atlanta
St. Louis	Kansas City
San Francisco	Columbus
Pittsburgh	Newark
Buffalo	Portland

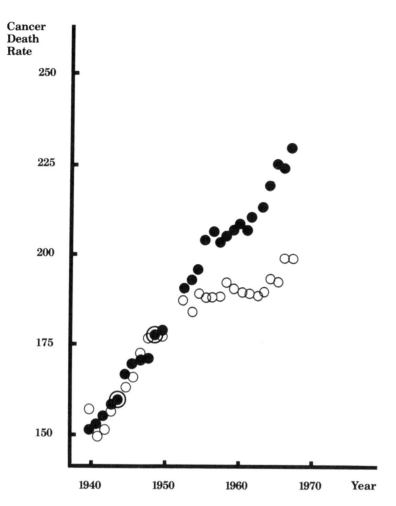

The vertical axis represents cancer death rate in terms of deaths per 100,000 population. The horizontal axis represents years from 1940 through 1970. The solid dots represent the year-by-year average cancer death rates of the ten largest cities fluoridated before 1957. The open circles represent the year-by-year average cancer death rate of the ten largest nonfluoridated cities — with comparable cancer death rates during the prefluoridation period (1940-1950) — which had not fluoridated before 1969. Fluoridation of the cites represented by solid dots began between 1952 and 1956. The data were obtained from standard government sources of vital statistics and census figures. (Data were not available for 1951 and 1952.) This graph represents one million cancer deaths, the cancer experience of 18 million Americans over 30 years.

This graph gives the year-by-year cancer death rates of both the fluoridated and nonfluoridated groups of cities: open circles represent the nonfluoridated cities and the solid dots represent the cities that were fluoridated after 1952.

Just by looking at this graph, one can see a strong association between fluoridation and cancer. Note how between 1940 and 1950, a time during which neither group of cities was fluoridated, the cancer death rates of both groups rose in a virtually identical fashion.

From 1952 to 1956, all of the experimental cities (represented by solid dots) had begun to fluoridate. As fluoridation was completed and continued year after year, the previous similarity in cancer death rates of the two groups of cities gave way to a noticeable divergency. The cancer death rate of the fluoridated group of cities increased drastically relative to that of the nonfluoridated group of cities.

By 1969, the fluoridated cities had an average cancer death rate of about 220-225 cancer deaths per 100,000 people, while the nonfluoridated cities had an average cancer death rate of 195-200 cancer deaths per 100,000 people. A comparison of the increase in cancer death rate of the fluoridated cities with the nonfluoridated cities showed a fluoride-linked increase of approximately 10% in only 13-17 years.

In 1976, these figures were checked and confirmed by the United States National Cancer Institute. However, some officials in the National Cancer Institute claimed that the increase in cancer death rates in fluoridated cities was due to changes in the age, sex, and racial composition in these cities.

When in the fall of 1977 these National Cancer Institute officials presented the data to support their claim before Representative L.H. Fountain's Congressional Subcommittee on Intergovernmental Relations, Dr. Yiamouyiannis pointed out that the National Cancer Institute officials had made an error in their calculations and had left out 80 to 90% of the relevant data. He pointed out further that when these errors and omissions were corrected, the National Cancer Institute's method confirmed the results of Drs. Burk and Yiamouyiannis showing a fluoride-linked increase in cancer deaths in the United States.

In 1977, Drs. Burk and Yiamouyiannis also conducted an

independent study of these same cities which showed that the fluoridation-linked increase observed could not be attributed to changes in the age, racial, or sex composition of the fluoridated and nonfluoridated populations. In this study, they determined the fluoridation-linked increase in cancer death rates of people of various ages. They found that the increase in cancer death rate observed in fluoridated cities occurred primarily in people ages 45-64 and 65 and over. This is apparent from the following table.

Age Group	FLUORIDATION-LINKED INCREASE IN CANCER DEATH RATE	
0-24	+0.4	cancer deaths per 100,000 population
25-44	+0.2	cancer deaths per 100,000 population
45-64	+8	cancer deaths per 100,000 population
65+	+35	cancer deaths per 100,000 population

The United States Centers for Disease Control, using a larger group of cities, confirmed the increased cancer death rates among people 45 years old and over living in fluoridated cities and presented a detailed breakdown of cancer death rates. These data are presented in the following table ('+' means the cancer death rate was higher in the fluoridated group, '-' means that the cancer death rate was lower in the fluoridated group).

FLUORIDATION-LINKED INCREASE IN CANCER DEATH RATE

Age Group	White Male	White Female	Nonwhite Male	Nonwhite Female
45-49	+	+	+	+
50-54	+	-	+	+
55-59	+	+	+	+
60-64	+	-	+	-
65-69	+	-	+	+
70-74	+	+	-	-
75-79	+	+	+	-
80-84	+	+	+	+
85+	+	+	-	+

The fact that fluoride affects older people is quite understandable. As people grow older, there is a decline in the DNA repair system and the immune system, the body's two major defense mechanisms against cancer. Thus, as people reach the age of 45 or more, the additional damage done by fluoride to an immune system and a DNA repair enzyme already weakened by age results in an increase in cancer death rates.

The claim of some National Cancer Institute officials that the fluoridation-linked increase in cancer deaths observed by Drs. Burk and Yiamouyiannis was due to changes in the age, race, and sex composition of the population was finally laid to rest in court cases in Pennsylvania and Illinois. In both cases, Drs. Burk and Yiamouyiannis met representatives of the National Cancer Institute head-on and were able to prove the fluoridation-cancer link to the court's satisfaction. As a result, both courts declared fluoridation a cancer threat and a threat to public health.

From the following table, which presents increases in age-, race-, and sex-adjusted cancer death rates of the fluoridated cities over and above those of the nonfluoridated cities, it can clearly be seen that there is substantial fluoridation-linked increase in cancer death rates.

FLUORIDATION-LINKED CANCER DEATHS PER 100,000 POPULATION CORRECTED FOR AGE, RACE, AND SEX

Before Initiation of Fluoridation	During Initiation of Fluoridation	After Initiation of Fluoridation		
1940-1949	1953-1956	1957-1960	1961-1964	1965-1968
0	4.3	7.3	7.8	10.3

The reason for age-race-sex adjustments of cancer death rates is not to necessarily get a more accurate picture of reality (such 'corrections' may actually distort the facts in the final analysis). It is a precautionary test to determine whether or not the increase in cancer death rate observed in fluoridated areas can be attributed to a combination of other factors, i.e. age, race, and sex.

The truth of the matter, according to Dr. Burk, is that age, race, and sex are only a few of the many factors which may contribute to or influence human cancer experience, some positively, others negatively. The 1940-1950 base-line figures presented on page 75 show that there was no difference in cancer death rates or their trends during this time. Since these cancer death figures are the result of the total of all known and unknown variables which influence cancer death rates, it is obvious that, whatever these variables were, their total effect on the cancer death rates of both groups of cities was virtually identical. Using a base-line control for known and unknown variables by initially comparing like with like, before introducing the factor to be tested, is basic to all scientific studies.

Dr. Burk concluded that, while adjustments, refinements, and corrections of the data on page 75 may provide interesting insights, the crude cancer death rates may well be the most accurate in the final analysis. To correct for a specific factor such as race when this item cannot be defined, quantified, and shown to be related to cancer can only lead to less accurate results.

To assure that the pattern of cancer death rates for nonfluoridated cities illustrated on page 74 was representative of large cities as a whole, Dr. Yiamouyiannis compared the cancer death rates of the ten largest fluoridated cities with the cancer death rates of the ten largest cities not fluoridated before 1957 with no requirement that the nonfluoridated cities have comparable cancer death rates to the fluoridated cities as of 1953. The first city of the nonfluoridated group to be fluoridated was fluoridated in 1965, so cancer death rates of this control group were only recorded until 1964.

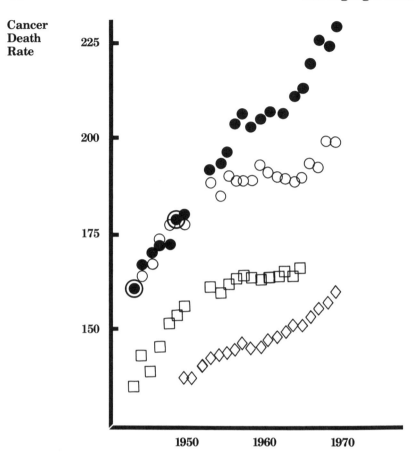

The vertical axis represents cancer death rate in terms of deaths per
100,000 population. The horizontal axis represents years from 1944
through 1970. The solid dots represent the year-by-year average
cancer death rates of the ten largest cities fluoridated before 1957.
The open circles represent the year-by-year average cancer death
rates of the 10 largest nonfluoridated cities with comparable cancer
death rates during the prefluoridation period (1940-1950) which had
not fluoridated before 1969. The open squares represent the year-by-
year average cancer death rates of the 10 largest cities not fluoridated before 1957. The open diamonds represent the year-by-year
average cancer death rates of the United States. Fluoridation of the
cities represented by solid dots began between 1952 and 1956. The
data were obtained from standard government sources of vital
statistics and census figures. (Data, other than national data, were
not available for 1951 and 1952). Since some of the cities in the
nonfluoridated group represented by open squares were fluoridated
in 1965, data for these cities as representative of nonfluoridated
cities was only recorded through 1964.

Fluoridated Cities	**Nonfluoridated Cities**
Chicago	New York
Philadelphia	Los Angeles
Baltimore	Detroit
Cleveland	Houston
Washington	Boston
Milwaukee	Dallas
St. Louis	New Orleans
San Francisco	San Antonio
Pittsburgh	San Diego
Buffalo	Seattle

The data presented in the graph includes the data previously presented on page 75 (solid dots and open circles) along with the year-by-year average cancer death rates of the new group of cities listed on this page (open squares) and the year-by-year cancer death rates of the United States (open diamonds).

As can be seen, the trends in cancer death rates of the two groups of nonfluoridated cities (open circles and open squares) are virtually identical. Comparison of the fluoridated cities with either group of nonfluoridated cities shows a substantial fluoridation-linked increase in cancer death rate. The year-by-year cancer death rates of the United States (open diamonds) show a cancer death rate trend initially comparable to that of the nonfluoridated cities. Note how the trend in the national cancer death rate increases as the United States becomes more fluoridated to a point where it falls between the cancer death rate trends of the fluoridated and nonfluoridated cities.

In other studies, Drs. Burk and Yiamouyiannis reported that fluoridated cities have higher cancer death rates than other cities in the surrounding geographical areas.

In yet another study, Drs. Burk and Yiamouyiannis looked at the cancer death rates of all cities east of the Mississippi River with populations of 10,000 or more and found a higher cancer death rate in fluoridated areas as compared to nonfluoridated areas.

As a result of their studies, Congressional Hearings were held in 1977. During the hearings, Drs. Yiamouyiannis and

Burk were able to show that the conflicting findings of U.S.
Public Health Service officials were due to the fact that they had
made mathematical errors and had left out 80-90% of the data
and that, when these errors and omissions were corrected, their
method of simultaneously adjusting for age, race, and sex
confirmed that 10,000 excess cancer deaths per year were linked
to water fluoridation in the U.S.

At the conclusion of these hearings, Rep. L. H. Fountain
stated: *"at the present time the carcinogenicity, or lack of carcinogenicity, of this substance is a question which remains unanswered"* and his committee instructed the U.S. Public Health
Service to conduct animal studies to determine whether or not
fluoride causes cancer. As a result, the U.S. Public Health
Service retained the Battelle Memorial Institute in Columbus,
Ohio to perform two studies, one on mice and another on rats.

Liver Cancer

On February 23, 1989, Battelle released the results of the mouse
study . The most significant finding of this study was the occurrence of an extremely rare form of liver cancer,
hepatocholangiocarcinomas, in fluoride-treated male and female
mice.

FLUORIDE-LINKED INCREASE IN
HEPATOCHOLANGIOCARCINOMAS

Fluoride in drinking water	Percent with hepatocholangiocarcinoma (animals with hepatocholangiocarcinoma/ total number of animals examined)	
	Males	**Females**
0 ppm	0% (0/79)	0% (0/80)
11 ppm	2% (1/50)	2% (1/52)
45 ppm	2% (1/51)	0% (0/50)
79 ppm	4% (3/80)	4% (3/80)

These cancers are so rare — that they are the first ones that Dr. John Toft (the mouse study project leader at Battelle Labs) had ever seen in his entire career of testing for cancer-causing substances. Among male mice, the odds of these results occurring by chance are less than 1 in 2,000,000. Among female mice, the odds of these results occurring by chance are less than 1 in 100,000. The odds of these results occurring by chance in both males and females are less than 1 in 200,000,000,000. In other words, this study shows clear evidence of the carcinogenic activity of fluoride in mice.

Oral Cancer

On April 11, 1989, Battelle released the results of the rat study. This study showed a dose-dependent relationship between oral squamous cell metaplasias (precancerous cells) and fluoride in both male and female rats.

FLUORIDE-LINKED INCREASE IN SQUAMOUS CELL METAPLASIAS

Fluoride in drinking water	Percent with oral metaplasias (animals with oral metaplasias/ total number of animals examined)	
	Males	Females
0 ppm	0% (0/80)	0% (0/79)
11 ppm	2% (1/50)	0% (0/50)
45 ppm	12% (6/50)	2% (1/50)
79 ppm	23% (18/80)	5% (4/80)

In addition, the Battelle rat study showed a dose-dependent relationship between fluoride and the oral tumors and cancers in male and female rats.

FLUORIDE-LINKED INCREASE IN
ORAL SQUAMOUS CELL TUMORS AND CANCERS

Fluoride in drinking water	Percent with oral tumors and cancers (animals with oral metaplasias/ total number of animals examined)	
	Males	Females
0 ppm	0% (0/80)	1% (1/79)
11 ppm	2% (1/50)	2% (1/50)
45 ppm	4% (2/50)	4% (2/50)
79 ppm	4% (3/80)	4% (3/80)

In response to the above results, the National Cancer Institute examined the incidence of oral cancer in fluoridated counties and nonfluoridated counties in the Iowa and Seattle areas for whites. The results of that study are tabulated below.

RATIOS OF ORAL CANCER RATES IN FLUORIDATED
AREAS TO ORAL CANCER RATES IN NONFLUORIDATED
AREAS (F/NF) BY DURATION OF FLUORIDATION FOR
THE IOWA AND SEATTLE AREAS AND BOTH AREAS
COMBINED FOR THE 1973-1987 SURVEY PERIOD.

Years of Exposure	Iowa F/NF	Iowa cases	Seattle F/NF	Seattle cases	Iowa+ Seattle
0-4	1.20	31	1.00	81	1.06
5-9	1.40	38	1.20	500	1.21
10-14	1.70	116	1.20	577	1.28
15-19	1.60	210	0.80	292	1.13
20+	1.60	848	—	—	1.60
All Periods	1.59	1243	1.11	1450	1.33

As can be seen from the above table, as exposure to fluoridation increases, so does the incidence of oral cancer. These data show at least a 33% to 50% increase in the incidence of the oral cancers in fluoridated areas. Nationally this would translate to 5000-7500 or more additional cases of oral and pharyngeal cancer per year as a result of fluoridation.

Bone Cancer

In 1989, Dr. Yiamouyiannis used the Freedom of Information Act to obtain carcinogenicity studies with sodium fluoride performed by Procter and Gamble and submitted to — but covered up by — the U.S. Public Health Service. These studies showed dose-dependent increases in ameloblastic squamous cell dysplasias (cell abnormalities which signal a transformation into a cancerous cell). These results were reported in the February 22, 1990 issue of the **Medical Tribune**. Additional studies by Procter and Gamble scientists confirmed the link between these precancerous growths and fluoride.

In another study, they concluded: *"There is clearly a compound[fluoride]-related increase in osteomas [bone tumors] in both male and female mice."* In addition, they found bone cancers and tumors in rats fed fluoride, but not in untreated rats.

In male rats exposed to higher fluoride levels, the Battelle study found osteosarcomas, rare cancers which are found in bone. No osteosarcomas were observed among females. These results are tabulated below.

FLUORIDE-LINKED OSTEOSARCOMAS

Fluoride in drinking water	Percent with osteosarcomas (animals with osteosarcomas/ total number of animals examined)
	Males
0 ppm	0% (0/80)
11 ppm	0% (0/50)
45 ppm	2% (1/50)
79 ppm	5% (4/80)

In 1991, the National Cancer Institute found that the incidence of osteosarcomas was about 50% higher in men 0-19 years of age exposed to fluoridated water as compared to those who were not.

In 1992, the New Jersey Department of Health published a study showing a substantial increase in the incidence of osteosarcoma in men under the age of 20 residing in fluoridated areas. Neither of these studies indicated a link between fluoride and bone cancer among women.

Thus, animal studies and human studies lead us to the conclusion that fluoride, while causing bone cancer in males, does not cause bone cancer in females. Biologically, this is reasonable, especially since the fluoride-linked bone cancer is noticed in males at a period of time in their life when they are shutting off bone growth by a process (the production of testosterone) that is different from the manner in which females shut off bone growth (estrogens). In 1983, Dr. K. C. Kanwar found that as little as 1 ppm fluoride inhibited testosterone synthesis under laboratory conditions.

Assuming that fluoride causes bone cancer in males but not females allows us to do a very definitive epidemiological study on humans. We can use females to serve as a control group for males residing in the same localities. By subtracting the bone cancer rate of females from that of males, we can eliminate the effect of factors that increase or decrease bone cancer in both males and females and confine our study to factors that only affect bone cancer in males.

In 1993, Dr. Yiamouyiannis completed this analysis of fluoride and bone cancer using bone cancer incidence data from the Surveillance, Epidemiology, and End Results (SEER) program of the National Cancer Institute (NCI) and from the New Jersey Department of Health, as well as mortality data from the National Cancer Institute. He found that:

1) the bone cancer incidence rate was as much as 0.95 new cases a year per 100,000 population higher in males under age 20 living in fluoridated areas;

2) the osteosarcoma incidence rate was 0.85 new cases a year per 100,000 population higher in males under age 20 living in fluoridated areas; and

3) for males of all ages, the bone cancer death rate and bone cancer incidence rate was as much as 0.23 and 0.44 cases higher per 100,000 population, respectively, in fluoridated areas.

These findings indicate that fluoridation is linked to about a 70% increase in bone cancer in men under age 20, and that a substantial part of this increase is due to an increase in osteosarcoma caused by fluoride.

Warning signs pointing out the potential of fluoridation to cause bone cancer are as old as fluoridation itself. Newburgh, New York was one of the first cities in the United States to be fluoridated. It was fluoridated in 1945 and a number of examinations were made on the children. The final report came out in 1956. Dr. John Caffey, a professor of clinical pediatrics at the College of Physicians and Surgeons, Columbia University, noted cortical defects in the bone x-rays of 13.5% of the children living in fluoridated Newburgh, compared to only 7.5% in the neighboring nonfluoridated town of Kingston. The difference was statistically significant and substantive. In another paper, Dr. Caffey had already noted that these bone defects were strikingly similar to that of osteogenic sarcoma, otherwise known as osteosarcoma. In making this observation, the National Academy of Sciences pointed out: *"While progression of cortical effects to malignancies has not been observed clinically, it would be important to have direct evidence that osteogenic sarcoma rates in males under 30 have not increased with fluoridation."* Well, as a matter of fact, they have increased, just as Dr. Caffey could have predicted 37 years ago.

Lung Cancer, Bladder Cancer, and Other Cancers

Dr. V. Cecilioni as well as Dr. N.N. Litvinov and co-workers from the USSR Academy of Medical Sciences and the Department of Air Hygiene in Moscow have linked lung cancer to high airborne fluoride levels.

In 1992, Dr. P. Grandjean and co-workers examined 423 cryolite workers with heavy exposure to fluoride and found 35 cases of lung cancer, 5 cases of cancer of the larynx, and 17 cases of urinary bladder cancer — rates that were higher than normal by 35% (for lung), 129% (for larynx), and 84% (for bladder). Cryolite contains about 50% fluoride. According to these researchers: *"Because this industrial cohort [i.e. group of workers] was exposed to high concentrations of fluoride dust, heavy respi-*

ratory exposure to fluoride may have contributed to the increased cancer risk."

WARNING: There is little doubt that fluoride (even down to and including the amounts used to fluoridate public drinking water) causes cancer.

1. The preponderance of evidence shows that fluoridation is causing an increase in bone cancer and deaths from bone cancer in human populations among males under age 20.

2. The increase in bone cancer attributable to fluoridation may all be due to an increase in osteosarcoma caused by fluoride.

3. The preponderance of evidence shows that fluoridation is causing an increase in oral cancer among human populations.

4. Since fluoride has been linked to bone and oral cancers in animals and humans, its biochemistry and its ability to inhibit the DNA repair enzyme system, to accelerate tumor growth rate, to inhibit the immune system, to cause genetic damage in a number of different cell lines, and to induce melanotic tumors, fibrosarcomas, hepatocholangiocarcinomas, and other tumors and cancers strongly indicate that fluoride has a generalized effect on increasing cancers overall.

5. According to our estimates, over 10,000 people in the United States die of cancer each year due to fluoridation of public drinking water.

Even Less Reliable Studies Show a Fluoridation-Cancer Link

In a 1992 study by Shupe and coworkers, a total of 10 male and 190 female cattle were subjected to low, moderate, and high fluoride exposures. Only those animals exposed to high fluoride exhibited cancers. One exhibited a squamous cell carcinoma and the other exhibited an 'undifferentiated' carcinoma. This rate of 2 fluoride-linked cancers per 87 animals is more than enough to be consistent with our figure of over 10,000 fluoridation-linked cancer deaths in the U.S. per year.

Other investigators have also published a number of studies concerning the effect of fluoridation on cancer death rate.

Dr. Donald Austin of the California Tumor Registry examined cancer death rates in California and found that people living in fluoridated areas had a cancer death rate which was 40% higher than those living in nonfluoridated areas.

Dr. John David Erickson of the Center for Disease Control examined the cancer death rates of all U.S. Cities with a population of 250,000 or more and found that in the year 1970, people in fluoridated areas experienced an age-sex-race corrected cancer death rate which was 4% higher than that of people in nonfluoridated cities.

Dr. John Knutson of the U.S. Public Health Service examined cancer death rates following fluoridation of Grand Rapids, Michigan and found a 22% increase in cancer death rate following fluoridation in contrast to the nonfluoridated control city of Muskegon, Michigan.

The problem with these studies (as well as other studies showing an increase in cancer death rates) is that many of them used a population too small to make any reliable conclusion as to whether fluoridation does or does not show an increase in cancer death rate in general. Other studies, such as the Erickson study, cannot be relied upon since they gave average cancer death rates for fluoridated and nonfluoridated cities for only one period (1969-1971) and thus did not allow for a time-trend analysis.

Effect of Fluoride on Total Mortality (Deaths from All Causes)

Deaths from all causes is 5% higher in fluoridated areas than in nonfluoridated areas according to figures from the Centers for Disease Control which were corrected for age, sex, and race.

Dr. Yiamouyiannis found that between 1950 and 1968, a comparison of the increase in age-sex-race corrected total death rate of the fluoridated cities with the nonfluoridated cities showed a fluoride-linked increase of 3-4% in about 15 years after fluoridation. In this study, he used the same cities that he had used for his cancer studies (see page 74).

This means that 30,000 to 50,000 deaths each year from various causes may now be attributable to fluoridation. This total includes the 10,000 to 20,000 deaths attributable to fluoride-induced cancer each year.

The fact that fluoride disrupts DNA repair enzyme activity, the fact that fluoride causes genetic damage, and the fact that fluoride causes cancer shows again that fluoride is directly accelerating the aging process.

Chapter 10

The Prime Target

It may be difficult at first to understand how a single substance like fluoride could cause such a wide variety of ill effects at a level as low as 1 part per million. The key is that fluoride at 1 part per million or even less interferes with the normal operation of a number of important enzymes.

Enzymes are proteins found in all living cells. They are responsible for catalyzing (or triggering) the chemical reactions that make life possible. These reactions lead to the breakdown of food to carbon dioxide, water, and urinary waste products; they produce the energy needed to support the life processes; they make possible the build-up of new tissues and the breakdown of old or unneeded tissues.

In the absence of enzymes, some of these reactions could not take place at body temperature, while others could not take place at all. For example, sugar is 'burned' in the body at 98.6° due to the action of enzymes, whereas sugar in a sugar bowl will not even begin to burn unless heated to over 250°, a temperature far above the boiling point of water and a temperature at which life cannot exist. The production of other substances in the body, such as DNA, RNA, and protein would be impossible without the involvement of enzymes.

The ability of fluoride to interfere with enzyme activity at 1 part per million or less is not a point of controversy. The United States National Academy of Sciences and the World Health Organization as well as others have published lists of enzymes that are inhibited at fluoride levels of 1 part per million or less. Remember, 1 part per million is the level of fluoride used to fluoridate public water systems. A partial list of enzymes inhibited by fluoride are presented in the following table.

ENZYME INHIBITION BY FLUORIDE AT
1 PART PER MILLION OR LESS

Enzyme	Fluoride Concentration	Percent Inhibition
Acetylcholinesterase	1ppm	61%
Glutamine Synthetase	1ppm	100%
DNA Repair Enzyme System	1ppm	50%
Lactoperoxidase	1ppm	50%
Pterin Deaminase	0.6ppm	50%
Alkaline Pyrophosphatase	0.4ppm	52%
dCMP Deaminase	0.3ppm	% not reported
Butyrylcholinesterase	0.3ppm	% not reported
ATPase	0.2 ppm	% not reported
Phosphomonoesterase	0.2 ppm	% not reported
Acid Glycerol Phosphatase	0.1ppm	% not reported

In an effort to down play the importance of this evidence, supporters of fluoridation have claimed that soft-tissue levels of fluoride (for example, the amount of fluoride in kidney, thyroid, spleen, etc.), even in people drinking fluoridated water, would never reach 1 part per million. Therefore, they maintained, the levels of fluoride necessary to inhibit these important enzymes would never be found in these tissues. This claim is incorrect, as can be seen in the table below.

ACCUMULATION OF FLUORIDE RESULTING FROM
FLUORIDE EXPOSURE

	Fluoride Concentrations in Organs of People	
	In 1939 Before Fluoridation Began in the U.S.	In 1960-65 After Fluoridation Began in the U.S.
Brain	0.53 ppm	1.5 ppm
Heart	0.51 ppm	1.8 ppm
Kidney	0.68 ppm	2.3 ppm
Liver	0.54 ppm	1.4 ppm
Lung	0.27 ppm	2.1 ppm
Spleen	0.28 ppm	1.8 ppm
Pancreas	not reported	1.7 ppm
Thyroid	not reported	4.0 ppm

This table shows that, in 1939, before fluoridation of public water supplies was begun in the United States, soft-tissue levels of fluoride were already found to contain about 0.5 part per million fluoride.

Between 1960 and 1965, soft-tissue fluoride levels were taken from the bodies of people who had lived in the greater Salt Lake City Area, which wasn't even fluoridated.[1] Their fluoride came only from foods and beverages shipped in from the neighboring fluoridated areas of San Francisco (fluoridated in 1952) and Denver (fluoridated in 1954), and from whatever industrial fluoride pollution of air and water there may have been in the vicinity. Even this indirect increase in exposure was enough to raise soft-tissue fluoride levels to 1.4-4.0 parts per million. More recent work by Dr. F. Geeraerts and co-workers from Vrije University in Brussels indicates a very active uptake of fluoride by the liver.

Additional enzymes which are inhibited at 2 parts per million fluoride, levels comparable to those found in the soft tissues of people exposed to fluoride, include: citrullinase, carbonic anhydrase, phosphatase, isocitric dehydrogenase, acid phosphatase, acetyl-CoA synthetase, lipase, and beta-glycerophosphatase.

It's quite evident that fluoride levels found in human tissues inhibit certain enzymes. The list of fluoride-sensitive enzymes presented in this chapter is by no means exhaustive.

It has been estimated that each cell contains thousands of different enzymes. It seems safe to say, based on the relatively few studies that have been done, that fluoride inhibits over 100 different enzymes in the soft tissues of people in fluoridated areas.

Thus, since enzymes are present in all living cells and are responsible for virtually all living processes, it is not surprising that fluoride can cause such a wide variety of ill-effects.

---

[1] Similar data for people living in fluoridated areas has not yet been reported.

Chapter 11

How Fluoride Works

While it has been known for some time that fluoride inhibits enzymes by binding to enzyme cofactors such as magnesium and phosphate, it was not until 1981 that chemists were able to explain how fluoride could chemically interact with enzymes themselves to cause enzyme inhibition.

In 1981, Dr. John Emsley and his co-workers at King's College in London found that fluoride forms very strong hydrogen bonds with groups of atoms called amides. As previously mentioned, enzymes are proteins. Proteins (enzymes) are large molecules composed of from about 100 to 1000 small molecular building blocks called amino acids (e.g. lysine, glutamic acid, tryptophan, etc.). The amino acids can be viewed as chain links, with each type of amino acid having its own characteristic structure. When these amino acid links are put together in a chain to form a protein, amides are formed by the junction of the links.

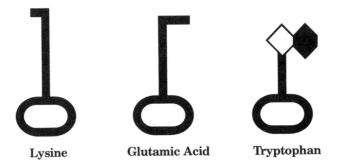

Lysine   **Glutamic Acid**   **Tryptophan**

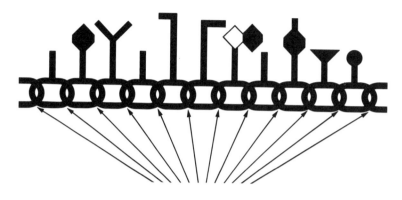

Amides

The different arrangements of these amino acids in a protein give rise to different proteins with differing sizes, differing enzymic activities, and differing susceptibilities to external conditions, such as exposure to fluoride (see the following illustration).

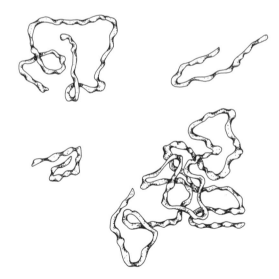

This figure illustrates 4 different protein chains. The smallest chain (lower left) consists of about 150 amino acid 'links'. The largest chain consists of about 1500 amino acid 'links'.

The characteristic shape of the protein is maintained by hydrogen bonds which tie certain of the protein's amide groups together. Dr. Emsley and co-workers showed that fluoride's hydrogen bond with amides is the second-strongest hydrogen bond ever found. Thus, fluoride has the ability to form hydrogen bonds with some of the protein's amide groups; as a result, fluoride disrupts the hydrogen bonds holding the protein in its normal shape.

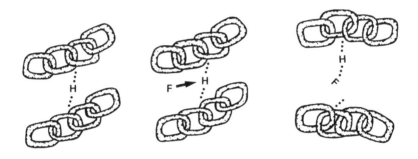

In this way, fluoride can disrupt the enzyme activity of proteins whose ability to trigger a reaction is highly dependent on a shape stabilized by these hydrogen bonds. Thus, in the illustration below, it can be seen how fluoride-disruption of protein structure can destroy the active site and thus the enzyme activity of proteins.

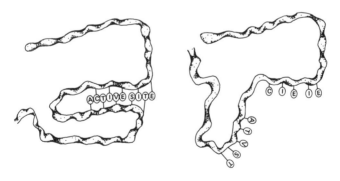

This in fact has been found by Dr. Edwards and co-workers from the University of California, San Diego by studying the effects of fluoride on the enzyme cytochrome c peroxidase. Based on the speed with which fluoride inhibited acetylcholinesterase, Drs. H.C. Froede and I.B. Wilson of the University of Colorado at Boulder suggested that fluoride inhibits the enzyme acetylcholinesterase *"by breaking and reforming hydrogen bonds."*

If the shape (or conformation) of the protein is greatly distorted by fluoride, the body's immune system will no longer be able to recognize the distorted protein as its own and will treat it instead as a foreign protein and attempt to destroy it. The immune response set off by the distorted protein can then be observed as an autoimmune allergic reaction, such as a skin reaction or gastrointestinal disturbance.

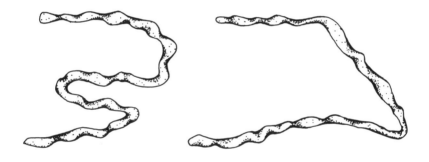

Normal Protein   **Distorted Protein**

Allergic or allergic-type responses to fluoride can result from the daily ingestion of the amount of fluoride found in one to two pints of artificially fluoridated water. These allergic responses have been reported in the literature and are listed in the ***Physicians' Desk Reference*** as well as the ***United States Pharmacopoeia***.

Hydrogen bonds are also responsible for stabilizing the structure of the genetic material of all animal cells, called DNA. DNA has a double-stranded structure which is stabilized by hydrogen bonds from the amides of one strand to those of the other. Disruption of the hydrogen-bonding of DNA provides still another mechanism by which fluoride might cause damage to the cell.

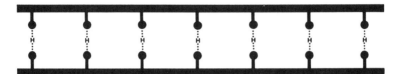

DNA strands connected by Hydrogen bonds

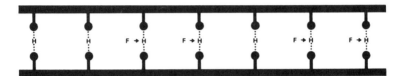

Fluoride attacking Hydrogen bonds

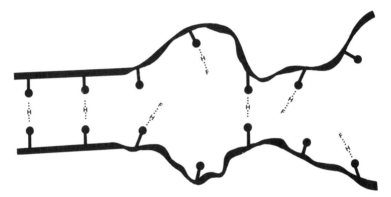

Disruption of Hydrogen bonds by Fluoride

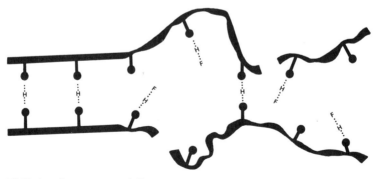

DNA (or chromosome) damage

The importance of Emsley's discovery of fluoride's strong hydrogen bonding with biologically important substances was noted by the editors of the journal, ***New Scientist***, who concluded: *"some of the charges that are laid at its door—genetic damage, birth defects, cancer and allergy response—may arise from fluoride interference after all."*

Since then, researchers from the University of California and the University of Colorado have confirmed that fluoride interference with hydrogen bonding causes a disruption of enzyme activity, as predicted in the first (1983) issue of this book.

It is important to understand that while it appears that fluoride causes a multiplicity of ill-effects, virtually all of these ill-effects can be traced to the effect of fluoride on enzymes or proteins, as well as a possible direct effect on the DNA molecule itself.

Chapter 12

How to Avoid Fluoride

In order to know how to avoid fluoride, one must know where to find it. In areas where the water is fluoridated, the largest amount of fluoride consumed comes from fluoride in the drinking water.

How to Avoid Fluoride from Fluoridated Water

In the home, the major part of this fluoride comes from water consumed directly from the tap if the water is fluoridated; water used to dilute fruit juices, fruit drinks, dry or concentrated infant formulas, etc.; water used to cook foods such as rice, spaghetti, hot cereals, beans, soups, etc.; water used to brew coffee and tea; water used to make bread, sprouts, etc. A copy of a comprehensive list of localities with fluoride in the water is available from the U.S. Centers for Disease Control, Atlanta, Georgia 30330; information as to whether a particular area is fluoridated can also be obtained by contacting the local water department.

A home water distiller provides the most reliable way to remove fluoride from the water in the home. The water from this unit should be used for drinking and for the preparation of all foods in the home. An alternate solution is to have distilled water delivered to the home. While spring water may also be used, care must be taken to be sure the spring water has a fluoride concentration of two-tenths (0.2) parts per million or less. Some spring waters are notoriously high in fluoride (Vichy and St. Yorre-Royale contain 8 ppm fluoride and consumption of these beverages has been linked to kidney disease and skeletal fluorosis). Most recently Beech-Nut, the company that sold colored sugar water to millions of unsuspecting Americans as apple juice to make a few more bucks, came out with a fluoridated bottle water for infants. Avoid it.

For those who are concerned that distilled water lacks minerals and that it may deplete the body of its minerals, it should be stressed that water is not a reliable source for minerals. In some cases, water may contain high magnesium/low calcium; in other areas it may contain low magnesium/high calcium or low magnesium/low calcium/high sodium or high arsenic/high fluoride/low magnesium. In order to receive a proper amount and balance of minerals, one must rely on a diet of fresh fruits, vegetables, nuts, seeds, and other natural products. These foods come from plants which have preselected those minerals which are necessary for the maintenance of life to the point where the plant has been able to produce the vegetation and(or) fruit which we eat.

Care should be taken to avoid beverages such as soft drinks, beers and wines, juice drinks and fruit juices from concentrate, etc. that have been bottled in fluoridated areas.

In a study of 43 ready-to-drink fruit juices by Dr. J. G. Stannard and co-workers, fluoride ion concentrations were examined. It was found that 42% of the samples had more than 1 ppm of fluoride. An analysis of 'Coke Classic' bottled in Chicago[2] showed that it contained 2.56 ppm fluoride; Diet Coke bottled in Chicago contained 2.96 ppm fluoride. Dr. P. T. Pang and co-workers found that mean daily fluoride intakes from beverages for North Carolina children 2-3, 4-6, and 7-10 years of age were 0.36, 0.54, and 0.60 mg, respectively.

Ideally, fruit juices from concentrate and fruit drinks should be avoided and replaced with 100% pure juices with no water added. Juices from concentrate are, by and large, a cheaper and inferior substitute. Fresh fruits are the ideal alternative.

A number of beers and wines are manufactured in fluoridated areas. Since manufacturers are required to list the location(s) where the bottling took place, one is able to determine whether the area is fluoridated and thus whether the wine or beer is fluoridated. Some widely known beers which are not fluoridated include Rolling Rock, Heineken, and Becks. Some beer manufacturers list a number of bottling plants, some fluoridated, some nonfluoridated, making it virtually impossible to determine whether or not the beer is fluoridated. If you are

---

[2] Analysis done by Coffey Labs in Portland Oregon.

fond of a particular beer or wine, it would be well worth your while to telephone the winery or brewery to ask about the product's fluoride content. Make sure you let them know what area of the country you live in so they can give you the accurate fluoride content of the product delivered to your area. If it turns out to be more than 0.4 parts per million fluoride, reject it.

Soft drinks should be avoided whether or not they are fluoridated, but if you are hooked on these health-menace beverages, you can use the same steps mentioned above for beers and wines to determine whether they are fluoridated.

Teas, even after being brewed with fluoride-free water, will contain about 1.2-2.4 ppm fluoride. According to the Tea Council (of Great Britain), the average person in Britain drinks 3.56 seven-ounce cups of tea per day. About 10% of the people don't drink tea. Thus the average tea drinker in Britain drinks closer to four cups (or 28 ounces) of tea per day and will consume 1-2 milligrams of fluoride even in nonfluoridated areas, about the same amount consumed by people living in fluoridated areas. It is not unusual for many in Britain to drink 7-8 7-oz. cups a day. Some drink as many as 15. The average person in the U.S. and Canada consumes less than one-half cup of tea per day. But whether you live in Britain, the U.S., or Timbuktu, if you drink tea, you will be getting large amounts of fluoride (most herbal teas are not a problem; however, some chamomiles have high fluoride concentrations). These amounts are large enough to cause dental fluorosis and all of the other harmful effects mentioned above.

Care should be taken to avoid food products from fluoridated areas in which water is a major constituent. In order to do this, make sure that you read the labels of the foods you buy and reject any food which lists water as one of the first three ingredients. (Food manufacturers are required to list the ingredients in decreasing order, i.e. the ingredient of highest content is listed first, the ingredient of next highest content is listed second, and so on.)

While at one time infant formulas were made with fluoridated water, they are not anymore. Concern among infant formula manufacturers led to their voluntary agreement (in 1980) to remove fluoride from the water used to manufacture infant formulas. Prior to 1980, almost all infant formulas were made with fluoridated water. (As early as 1974, Dr. Yiamouyiannis alerted the FDA to the dangers fluoride presents to infants. Because babies consume such a tremendous amount of liquid relative to their weight, he noted, heart damage as well as other complications might occur. He cited numerous studies in support of his charges.) Mother's milk, the beverage of choice, contains only 0.01-0.05 ppm fluoride, a level below that found in any other food. This is nature's way of protecting the infant from fluoride damage.

How to Avoid Fluoride from Other Products

Other sources of fluoride around the home include fluoridated toothpastes, mouthwashes, vitamin tablets, and vitamin drops. These products should be immediately discarded and replaced with nonfluoridated products.

Dentists routinely offer to give fluoride treatments. These treatments should be refused. In cases where the dentist becomes arrogant, seek another dentist.

Three sources of fluoride exposure exist in schools: 1) A number of schools around the country have adopted fluoride mouthrinse programs. 2) If the school is in a fluoridated area, the drinking water is fluoridated, and in some rural schools, 5-7 parts per million is added to the school drinking water! 3) Finally, some schools spread fluoride around the cafeteria areas to kill rats, mice, roaches, and silverfish, thus causing a risk of food contamination or inhalation of the fluoride powder.

To avoid these exposures, parents should refuse to sign permission slips for the school mouthrinse programs and see that these programs, as well as school fluoridation programs are stopped. They should also make sure that fluoride, which is not biodegradable, is no longer used in schools as a pesticide and rodenticide.

Even those promoting fluoridation are beginning to come out against the use of fluoride products. What follows is a sorry history of how they have allowed millions of children to be poisoned by fluoride tablets and drops through their ignorance and unwillingness to admit they were wrong in a timely manner.

In 1977, the *Fluoride Symposium of the 143rd Annual Meeting of the American Association for the Advancement of Science* and again in 1978, the *Journal of the American Dental Association* reported that 0.5-mg fluoride supplements were causing dental fluorosis. But nothing was done about it. In the *1978 Physicians' Desk Reference* (p. 1637), the following statement with regard to fluoride supplements was still made: *"A daily fluoride intake of 0.5 mg from birth to age three years . . . is recommended."*

In the *1983 Physicians' Desk Reference* (p. 1977) the above statement with regard to fluoride supplements was modified: *"In communities with less than 0.3 ppm fluoride in the water supply, the recommended dosage is 0.25 mg daily between birth and two years of age."*

Apparently, the visible devastation of the teeth of 25,000,000 to 30,000,000 people in the United States and Canada with dental fluorosis is having an effect on the Canadian Dental Association. In 1992, it issued its 'Proposed Fluoride Guidelines' which now states: *"Fluoride supplements should not be recommended for children less than three years old."*

Exceptionally high rates of dental fluorosis are being observed among children consuming fluoride tablets. In Amsterdam, 74% of the children participating in a fluoride program developed dental fluorosis as a result of the consumption of fluoride tablets.

The only reason that these fluoridation promoters are attacking fluoride supplements is that fluoride poisoning is becoming pandemic, and by placing the blame elsewhere, they can try to escape responsibilty for the damage water fluoridation has done, and is doing, to tens of millions of North Americans.

Warning: People using fluoride tablets for the treatment of osteoporosis should stop using them immediately.

How to Avoid Fluoride When Eating Out

When eating out in fluoridated areas, water as well as foods made with water such as soups, beans, rice, pasta, soft drinks, and coffee or tea should be avoided. Orders should consist of meats, salads, baked potatoes, dairy products and other foods which are not made with water or which do not tend to soak up water while cooking.

Special Considerations

Some foods are high in fluorides even in the absence of added fluoride from the water. For example, as mentioned above, some tea leaves are notoriously high in fluoride, and even tea made in distilled water can result in a beverage containing 1-2 parts per million of fluoride or more. Foods which are naturally low in fluoride include fresh fruits, vegetables, whole grain cereals, nuts, meat, and dairy products. Ready-to-eat cereals, such as corn flakes and grape nuts, are notoriously high in fluoride.

People living in the vicinity of aluminum, phosphate, steel, clay, glass, enamel, and many other types of manufacturing plants are exposed to high levels of fluoride in the air. People employed in these industries can have an even higher exposure. In order to avoid this exposure, moving or seeking employment elsewhere is the only immediate alternative. The decision is a decision between a person's health or a better-paying job — a decision between staying in a hazardous area or moving. It is not a new decision. Coal miners, knowing that they are killing themselves with black lung disease, have opted to sell their health for a larger paycheck. However, people who consider their health of primary importance should try to move out of these areas and out of these jobs until manufacturers are able and willing to apply technology to clean up the fluoride pollution problems on the job and in the surrounding areas.

Food grown in these polluted areas, especially fruits, vegetables, and grains, become contaminated with fluoride. This leads to higher fluoride intakes. Additionally, fruits, vegetables, and grains grown with low-grade fluoride-contaminated phosphate fertilizers will pick up a higher fluoride content. It has been found that the use of cheap, fluorine-containing fertilizers can result in a 6- to 12-fold increase in dietary fluoride. Some foods are also contaminated with fluoride-containing pesticides. Modern food distribution, because it brings foods in from a wide range of different geographical areas, prevents this from being as serious as it is for people who get most of their food either from these polluted areas or from areas using low-grade phosphate fertilizers.

Chapter 13

The First Fable:
Fluoride is Essential

$\mathbf{P}$eople who have heard that reducing fluoride in their diets can lead to some type of nutritional deficiency should be aware that there is no evidence that fluoride in any amount is a necessary nutritional ingredient. In 1971, the U.S. National Academy of Sciences reviewed a number of studies on the subject and concluded that fluoride had not been shown to be an essential nutrient. (These studies on the essentiality of fluoride, as is true of all studies attempting to determine essentiality, confined themselves primarily to the measurement of weight gain and reproductive function, and did not deal with the biochemical disturbances and pathological effects of fluoride discussed previously in this book.)

The National Academy of Sciences outlined the tests which a substance or element must pass before being called an essential nutrient: *"First, it should be possible to demonstrate repeated and significant responses in growth or health to dietary supplements of the element and to the element alone; second, it should be possible to develop a deficiency state on diets that lack the element but that are otherwise adequate and satisfactory. Such diets should contain all other known dietary essentials in adequate amounts."* Regarding the claim that fluoride might reduce tooth decay, the Academy points out: *"That in itself is no indication of fluorine essentiality, inasmuch as caries incidence depends on many factors, and many persons with perfectly sound dentition have had only minimal exposure to fluoride."*

One of the studies referred to by the National Academy of Sciences in support of their conclusion that fluoride is not an essential nutrient was done by Drs.. Richard L. Maurer and Harry G. Day of the Department of Chemistry at Indiana University in Bloomington. Drs. Maurer and Day purified all dietary ingredients to produce a diet that contained about 0.007 parts per million fluoride, which is extremely low. They raised rats on this diet and double-distilled water through four generations, comparing them to rats fed the same diet but given 2 parts per million fluoride in their drinking water. Drs. Maurer and Day pointed out: *"Under the extremely rigorous conditions of this study, fluorine was not found to have any influence on the growth and well-being of rats. There were not even any grossly detectable dental defects. Thus it is justifiable to conclude that under some conditions, fluorine may not have any value in nutrition or even in the maintenance of dental health."*

Another of the studies referred to by the National Academy of Sciences in support of their conclusion that fluoride is not a dietary essential was one by Dr. A.R. Doberenz and other researchers at the University of Arizona in Tucson. These researchers developed a diet that contained even less fluoride— under 0.005 parts per million. Still, they were unable to notice any difference in general health between rats fed that diet and rats fed the same diet plus 2 parts per million fluoride in their drinking water.

Since that time, only two studies have claimed that fluoride is an essential nutrient and both have been thoroughly discredited.

The first of these is a study by Drs. Klaus Schwarz and Robert Milne of the Veterans Administration Hospital in Long Beach, California. In 1972, they reported that in rats fed a synthetic diet containing low amounts (0.04-0.46 parts per million) of fluoride and kept in incubators to eliminate airborne fluoride, the addition of fluoride stimulates growth. A brief look at the control animals with fluoride in the diet used by Drs. Schwarz and Milne (see the following figure) indicates that these animals were too sick to yield meaningful results.

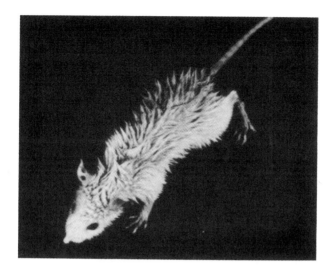

In 1974, Drs. F.H. Nielsen and A.A. Sandstead from the U.S. Department of Agriculture Human Nutrition Laboratory reviewed the study by Drs. Schwarz and Milne. They pointed out that both groups of animals (with and without fluoride) were too sick for the data to be reliable. They also pointed out that the differences in weight gain between the fluoride and nonfluoride groups were small and that: *"Others have not been able to confirm this finding even though they have fed diets containing even less fluorine."*

The second study that tried to show that fluoride is an essential nutrient was published in 1973 by Drs. H.H. Messer, Wallace Armstrong and Leon Singer of the University of Minnesota. Female mice were fed a low-fluoride diet (0.1 to 0.3 parts per million fluoride) plus drinking water containing either 0, 50, 100 or 200 parts per million fluoride. The mice given the two higher levels of fluoride became sick or died. Mice on water containing 50 parts per million fluoride produced litters sooner than did mice receiving no fluoride in their drinking water, but the absence of fluoride in the drinking water had no effect on growth rate or litter size.

The researchers reported that the low-fluoride mice developed signs of fluoride deficiency, with a progressive development of infertility in two successive generations. However, they did not take into consideration dietary levels of other trace elements. Dr. Messer acknowledged, at the 1974 Symposium on Trace Element Metabolism in Animals, that the diet of the mice contained only marginal concentrations of iron. The National Academy of Sciences points out that when testing for essentiality of a substance: *"Such diets should contain all other known dietary essentials in adequate amounts."* The experiments of Dr. Messer and co-workers did not meet this requirement.

This experiment was repeated in 1976 by Drs. S. Tao and J.W. Suttie of the University of Wisconsin, only this time the animals were provided with adequate concentrations of iron. The researchers reported that differences in reproduction between the high-and low-fluoride groups disappeared. Drs. Tao and Suttie explained: *"The results of the present study suggest that the apparent essentiality of fluoride previously observed was due to pharmacological (drug-like) effect of fluoride in improving iron utilization in a diet marginally sufficient in iron. The data do not support the previous claims of an essential role of fluoride in reproduction."*

Furthermore, nobody would ever suggest giving the 50 parts per million fluoride used in the experiments of Dr. Messer and co-workers, to humans as a 'nutritional supplement' (50 ppm fluoride is the level of fluoride dumped into the water during the Annapolis disaster, see Chapter 2).

The studies of Dr. Messer and his co-workers are directly contradicted by the research of Drs. S.W.J. Van Reensburg and W.H. De Vos from the Veterinary Research Institute in Onderstepoort, South Africa. These investigators looked at the calving rates of cows treated with water containing fluoride at 5, 8, and 12 parts per million (remember: some schools are presently adding 5-7 parts per million fluoride to the drinking water). As can be seen in the following diagram, fluoride produces a sharp decrease in the ability of cows to reproduce normally, and this decrease is greater among cows that are exposed to greater levels of fluoride.

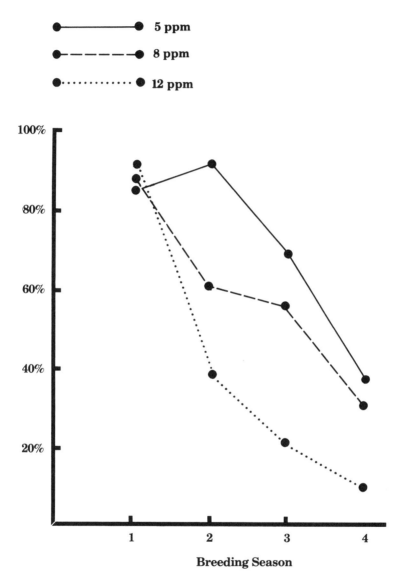

Calving rate of cows on three of levels of fluoride intake: 5, 8, and 12 parts per million.

Drs. Van Reensburg and De Vos pointed out: *"It is significant that evidence of interference with reproduction was shown
long before there were any symptoms of ill health, inappetence
(loss of appetite) or mottling of the teeth. . .not one of the animals
showed signs of poor health or loss of appetite up to the end of the
fourth breeding season, though erosion, pitting and mottling of
the teeth became increasingly evident."*

More recent laboratory studies have shown that 1 part per
million fluoride leads to depressed testosterone synthesis.
Additional studies have shown that fluoride treatments lead to a
depression of testicular and spermatozoid function in males and
a loss of fertility in females.

The October 12, 1984 issue of the **Wall Street Journal** in a
front-page story pointed out: *"In recent years, infertility specialists have seen a marked increase in the number of couples unable
to conceive. . .At the same time physicians note, the average
sperm count among men is decreasing. Toxic environmental
pollution is thought to be a culprit."*

Other Considerations

In 1974, Drs. C.W. Weber and B.L. Reid at the University of
Arizona again conducted research to determine whether fluoride
was an essential nutrient. They found no 'beneficial' effects on
mice supplemented with fluoride as compared with low-fluoride
mice through six generations, even though bone fluoride levels
showed that the higher doses of fluoride were getting into the
animals' bodies.

To be an essential element, a substance must participate in
some physiological function. For example, magnesium serves as
a cofactor to make certain enzymes function and sulfur serves to
stabilize the structure of enzymes. The effect of fluoride is just
the opposite. It disrupts the function of normal metabolism.

Probably the most disruptive effect of fluoride is its interference with the use of oxygen by cells in the body. Fluoride inhibits the normal use of oxygen and has been shown to depress the
synthesis of an energy-producing substance called ATP.
Enzymes called cytochromes, cytochrome oxidases, and cytochrome peroxidases are responsible for the proper utilization of

oxygen to produce ATP.

In 1984, it was shown that fluoride forms hydrogen bonds with an iron-containing enzyme called cytochrome c peroxidase. This enzyme is involved in the use of oxygen for 'burning' various foods. As little as two-tenths part per million fluoride is calculated to result in a 50% bonding of fluoride to the enzyme. In so binding to the enzyme, fluoride would be expected to interfere with the proper utilization of oxygen.

Dr. Thomas L. Poulos, one of the coauthors of the report, pointed out that because of the similarity in the configuration around the iron in this enzyme and another enzyme called cytochrome oxidase, he would expect fluoride to also bind with cytochrome oxidase. Not only would this interfere with oxygen utilization and ATP production, it also explains the reason fluoride induces the unnecessary and destructive production of superoxide free radicals (O_2^-) (see Chapter 3). (Normally the cytochromes catalyze the production of water from oxygen and electrons (e^-) derived from food, i.e. $O_2 + 4e^- + 4H^+ \longrightarrow 2H_2O$. By disrupting oxygen metabolism at the first step, fluoride can induce the formation of superoxide, i.e. $O_2 + e^- \longrightarrow O_2^-$).

In summary, fluoride is not an essential nutrient. Not one person has ever been found with a fluoride deficiency. Quite simply put, fluoride is a poison. And even though some essential nutrients such as Vitamin A and copper are poisonous at higher levels, neither Vitamin A nor copper has been used to kill rats, cockroaches, and silverfish. Fluoride is routinely used as a rodenticide and insecticide.

Chapter 14

The Second Fable:
Fluoride Reduces
Tooth Decay

"If one wishes to be free from toothache, one should eat a whole mouse twice a month or wash the mouth out three times a year with the blood of a tortoise."

Pliny, circa 50 A.D.

As was noted in Chapter 5, fluoride is responsible for mottling of the teeth, particularly in undernourished children. Dr. Gerald J. Cox of the Mellon Institute was aware of fluoride's mottling effect. However, in 1937, he concluded, *"It is possible that fluorine is specifically required for the formation of teeth."* Keep in mind that Dr. Cox was with the Mellon Institute which was and is associated with the Aluminum Company of America (ALCOA), a major fluoride polluter.

Also in 1937, Dr. Cox addressed the 'Open Forum on Causes and Control of Dental Caries' and spoke of *"evidence . . . that there is an optimum amount of fluorine essential for good tooth formation."* That evidence was not given at the forum. Dr. Cox went on to say, *"The optimum, of course, is below that which causes mottled enamel."* In the 1938 ***Journal of the American Dental Association***, Dr. Cox stated that *"fluorine is responsible for . . . increased resistance to caries . . . the case should be regarded as proved."*

Just where did this proof come from? Suddenly, fluoride was no longer a poison to be wary of, but the important factor in preventing tooth decay.

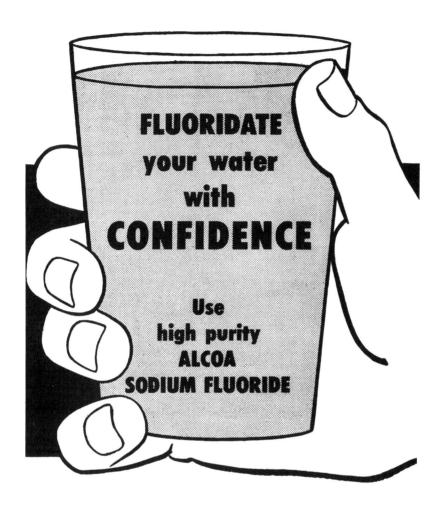

FROM the *Journal of the American Water Works Association*

Three lines of evidence were published in 1938 to fulfill the 'prophecy' of Dr. Cox. They included: a study claiming that sound teeth contained more fluoride than decayed teeth; a laboratory study claiming that the offspring of female rats fed fluoride had less tooth decay; and a study claiming that people in high-natural-fluoride areas had less tooth decay than those in low-fluoride areas.

Fluoride Makes the Teeth Stronger?

In 1938, Drs. Wallace Armstrong and P.J. Brekhus from the University of Minnesota Department of Biochemistry published a study in which they claimed that the enamel of sound teeth had a significantly greater fluoride content than the enamel of teeth with cavities. But 25 years later, Dr. Armstrong was forced to admit that these results were false. In a follow-up study in 1963, Dr. Armstrong found no difference in the fluoride contents of the enamel of sound and decayed teeth.

Animal Studies

One would think that a chemical ought to be proven beneficial before being used on the general population. Common sense would dictate that the proof be obtained through controlled laboratory experiments before subjecting a large part of the human population to the substance. Not so in the case of fluoride. Laboratory tests, conducted to determine whether fluoride reduces tooth decay when added to the drinking water at a concentration of 1 part per million, have failed to produce positive results.

Consider these laboratory findings:

Dr. Cox claimed in 1938 that he had found that adding fluoride to the drinking water reduced tooth decay. In 1939, he published the results of his study. In this study, 10 to 40 parts per million fluoride were added to the diet of pregnant rats and tooth decay was determined in their offspring which were killed after 8 weeks. From the results of the study, which are summarized below, it is difficult to see any beneficial effect from the addition of fluoride to the drinking water.

TOOTH DECAY RATE IN OFFSPRING OF PREGNANT RATS FED FLUORIDE

	Fluoride Added to the Diet (ppm)			
	0	10	20	40
Cavities Between Teeth	11	10	13	8
Cavities on the Biting Surfaces of Molar Teeth	17	17	20	14

Studies done since then show that the amount of fluoride used to fluoridate public water systems does not reduce tooth decay under laboratory conditions.

Drs. J.L. Hardwick and D.M. Bunting of the Turner Dental School in Manchester, England examined the effect of fluoridation on tooth decay in rats. Reporting their findings in the *Journal of Dental Research* in 1971, they said, *"Changes in the number of lesions were not significant with 1 or 2 part per million fluoride supplementation."* In other words, fluoride did virtually nothing to reduce tooth decay in rats in this experiment.

In 1962, Dr. Edward A. Sweeney and co-workers at the Harvard School of Dental Medicine reported in the *Journal of Dental Research* that fluoride had little effect on tooth decay rates of laboratory rats. However, the amount of fluoride present in the bones of the animals was significantly greater among the fluoride groups. This shows that the animals in the fluoride groups did in fact take in more fluoride. Yet, as the following table indicates, it made little difference with regard to tooth decay.

THE EFFECT OF FLUORIDE IN DRINKING WATER
ON TOOTH DECAY IN RATS

	Number of Decayed Molar Teeth	Total Number of Decayed Teeth	Bone Fluoride (ppm)
Group #1			
0 ppm fluoride	5.4	6.2	96
1 ppm fluoride	6.6	8.8	137
Group #2			
0 ppm fluoride	6.9	10.3	41
1 ppm fluoride	5.8	9.3	89
Group #3			
0 ppm fluoride	5.2	8.4	-
1 ppm fluoride	5.5	8.1	-
Average			
0 ppm fluoride	5.8	8.3	
1 ppm fluoride	6.0	8.7	

More recently, Dr. Spuller and co-workers from Ohio State University reported 4.2 caries per rat for animals receiving 0 ppm fluoride in their drinking water and 3.1 caries per rat for animals receiving 1 ppm fluoride in their drinking water, but found that in rats receiving 0 and 1 ppm fluoride in Coca Cola, caries rates were 8.2 and 10.0, respectively. Taken together, these data do not show that 1 ppm fluoride in the water has any effect on tooth decay under laboratory conditions.

But Spuller's group maintained that the reduction in tooth decay they observed at 1 ppm is significant, pointing out that, in follow-up studies, they got identical reductions in tooth decay compared to controls whether they used 0.25 ppm fluoride in the drinking water, which gave them a 20% reduction in caries rates, or 1 ppm fluoride in the drinking water, which gave them a 19% reduction in caries rates. Even at face value, their results do not indicate that fluoridation of drinking water reduces tooth decay, because most nonfluoridated waters already have fluoride concentrations in the 0.25 ppm range. Furthermore, their studies do not rule out the possibility that 0.1 ppm or lower concentrations of fluoride would have the same 'caries-inhibiting' effects.

There are no other laboratory studies on rats or any other animal that either show or even claim to show that 1 ppm fluoride in the drinking water is effective in reducing tooth decay. The United States Public Health Service acknowledges this, but claims that rat dentition is not suitable for testing the decay-reducing potential of fluoride. However, USPHS researchers were the first to use rats to see if fluoride levels comparable to those currently used to fluoridate drinking water could reduce tooth decay.

Tooth Decay Lower in High Fluoride Areas?

In 1938, Dr. H. Trendley Dean, the first director of the National Institute of Dental Research, claimed to have found that fluoride in the drinking water was responsible for a reduction in tooth decay in children. He said that only 30 percent of 9-year-olds living in areas with what he called a low natural fluoride content of 0.6 to 1.5 parts per million in the drinking water (Pueblo, Colo.; Junction City, Kans.; and East Moline, Ill.) had decay-free permanent teeth. In contrast, he pointed out that 60 percent of the children living in areas with a higher natural fluoride content of 1.7 to 2.5 parts per million in the water (Monmouth, Ill.; Galesburg, Ill.; and Colorado Springs, Colo.) had decay-free permanent teeth. However, an examination of his data shows that claims attributing lower tooth decay rates to fluoride don't hold up. From the following data, it is difficult to discern any beneficial effect from higher levels of fluoride in the water.

EFFECT OF FLUORIDE ON TOOTH DECAY RATES IN HUMANS

Locality	Fluoride parts per million	Percent of Children with Decay-Free Permanent Teeth	Percent of Children with Dental Fluorosis
Pueblo, Colo.	0.6	37	2.4
Junction City, Kans.	0.7	26	1.7
East Moline, Ill.	1.5	11	24.5
Monmouth, Ill.	1.7	55	42.1
Galesburg. Ill.	1.8	56	35.1
Colorado Springs, Colo.	2.5	41	67.6

If Dr. Dean were trying to point out that 1.7 to 2.5 parts per million fluoride were necessary for cavity prevention, he would also have had to admit that these same levels of fluoride produced mottling in 40 to 70 percent of the children. In a subsequent study in 1942, Dean grouped Moline, Ill. with high-fluoride areas because in this study, instead of having the highest tooth decay rate, it had the lowest.

In a 1970 follow-up study of the findings of Dr. Dean, Drs. Fred L. Losee and Basil G. Bibby re-examined some of Dean's figures and showed that, in cases where the tooth decay rates of 12- to 14-year-old children went down as fluoride levels in the drinking water went up, the reduction in tooth decay could as easily have been attributed to strontium and/or boron as to fluoride. To back up this statement they presented data from the following communities in Illinois.

CORRELATIONS OF TOOTH DECAY RATES WITH FLUORIDE AND OTHER MINERALS

City	Strontium parts per million	Boron parts per million	Fluoride parts per million	Decayed Missing, & Filled Permanent Teeth
Galesburg	2.0	0.5	1.9	2.36
Aurora	1.0	0.3	1.2	2.81
Joliet	0.5	0.5	1.3	3.23
Oak Park	0.1	0.02	0.0	7.22
Quincy	0.03	0.01	0.1	7.06
Waukegan	0.02	0.02	0.0	8.10

Dean's studies have been widely cited by fluoridation promoters because they supposedly proved the benefits of fluoride. As a matter of fact, what they really showed was that fluoride has little if any effect on tooth decay. The results of other researchers also show no apparent effect.

Dr. Eugene Zimmerman and co-workers from the National Institute of Dental Research reported on a 10-year study of Bartlett, Texas (8 parts per million fluoride) and Cameron, Texas (0.4 parts per million fluoride). Their report, published in a 1955 issue of the *Journal of the American Dental Association*, noted that the incidence of tooth decay was *"examined statistically and no significant difference was found between the Bartlett and Cameron residents."*

A slightly earlier study in Arizona likewise found no significant difference in tooth decay rates between high- and low-fluoride areas. Dentist Donald J. Galagan conducted the study on 12- to 14-year-olds. He published the results in the *Journal of the American Dental Association* in 1953. His data (which are reproduced in the following table) indicate, that while dental fluorosis (mottling) increased and became more severe as the fluoride concentration in the water increased, no reduction in the number of decayed, missing and filled teeth per child could be observed.

EFFECT OF FLUORIDE ON TOOTH DECAY RATES IN HUMANS

	Fluoride (ppm)	Number of Children	Decayed, Missing, & Filled Teeth Per Child	Number of Children	Percent With Dental Fluorosis
Yuma	0.4	29	2.45	82	4
Tempe	0.5	45	2.82	113	10
Tucson	0.7	167	3.48	316	17
Chandler	0.8	42	2.45	95	19
Casa Grande	1.0	22	2.00	50	48
Florence	1.2	34	3.56	70	56

In probably the largest study of tooth decay in areas with various natural levels of fluoride in the drinking water, Dr. Yoshitsugu Imai of the Tokyo Medical and Dental University examined more than 20,000 students, grades 1 through 6. In 1972, he reported the results of this study. He found a higher percentage of students with tooth decay in areas with fluoride levels of 0.4 parts per million or more in the drinking water than in areas with 0.2 to 0.39 parts per million in the drinking water.

The question now is: 'Does all this mean fluoride doesn't reduce tooth decay?'

Well, numerous attempts have been made to show that the amount of fluoride used to fluoridate public water systems reduces tooth decay under laboratory conditions. Still — and the U.S. Center for Disease Control and the British Ministry of Health admit this — no laboratory study has ever shown that the amount of fluoride added to drinking water is effective in reducing tooth decay. Furthermore, they admit that there are no epidemiological studies on humans showing that fluoridation reduces tooth decay that meet the minimum requirements of scientific objectivity. These requirements are referred to by scientists as blind or double-blind design, in which neither examiner nor patient know who is in the test group and who is in the control group. This type of study is necessary to eliminate examiner-patient bias. It also helps to prevent misleading results. For instance, tooth decay rates among U.S. children living in some fluoridated areas are more than twice as high as those living in other areas that are nonfluoridated. And comparisons showing the opposite can also be found. Blind and double-blind design helps assure an unbiased selection of areas so that reliable results can be obtained.

The Fluoridation Experiment Begins

The studies of Dr. Cox, Dr. Armstrong, and Dr. Dean hardly proved the benefits of fluoride. Yet, it was on the basis of these studies that fluoridation of public water supplies began.

Grand Rapids, Michigan, the first city reported to be fluoridated, began to add fluoride to the drinking water on January 25, 1945; Muskegon, Michigan was selected as a control (nonfluoridated) city. The study was originally designed to last for at least 10 years, but five years after fluoridation began, it was observed that the tooth decay rates of both artificially fluoridated Grand Rapids and nonfluoridated Muskegon had decreased, as can been seen from the following table derived from studies originally published by USPHS scientists.

DECAYED, MISSING, AND FILLED
PERMANENT TEETH (DMFT) PER CHILD

Age	Grand Rapids (fluoridated)			Muskegon (nonfluoridated)		
	1944-45	1949-50	Change	1944-45	1949-50	Change
5	0.11	0.03	-0.08	0.06	0.14	+0.08
6	0.78	0.38	-0.40	0.81	0.63	-0.18
7	1.89	0.76	-1.13	1.99	1.43	-0.56
8	2.94	2.16	-0.78	2.81	2.58	-0.23
9	3.90	2.48	-1.42	3.81	3.88	+0.07
10	4.92	3.56	-1.36	4.91	4.44	-0.47
11	6.41	4.69	-1.72	6.32	5.93	-0.39
12	8.07	7.02	-1.05	8.66	7.21	-1.45
13	9.73	8.11	-1.62	9.98	9.52	-0.46
14	10.94	8.90	-2.04	12.00	11.08	-0.92
15	12.48	11.80	-0.68	12.86	10.32	-2.54
16	13.50	11.83	-1.67	14.07	12.51	-1.56
Average	6.31	5.14	-1.16	6.52	5.81	-0.72

Thereafter Muskegon was dropped as a control city and the only result publicized was that the tooth decay rate in Grand Rapids decreased after fluoridation. (It is interesting that this experimental 'abortion' took place at the precise time that the fluoridation bandwagon began rolling (see Chapter 16).

The major fluoridation study in Britain, carried out by the British Ministry of Health, also failed to show a significant reduction in tooth decay from fluoridation. The average number of decayed, missing and filled permanent teeth per child was reported for 8-, 9-, and 10-year-olds for the years 1955-56, when fluoridation began, and for 1967. Out of five populations studied, two groups (designated F1 in the table below) received drinking water containing 1 part per million fluoride for the entire period of time. Another group (designated PF) received drinking water containing 1 part per million fluoride for three years, a fourth group (F.7) received drinking water containing 0.7 part per million fluoride for the entire time period, and the last group (NF) received drinking water containing no added fluoride for the entire time period. From the tabulated results below, it is difficult to see any beneficial effect from fluoride.

TOOTH DECAY (THE NUMBER OF DECAYED, MISSING & FILLED PERMANENT TEETH PER CHILD)

Area	1955/56	1967	Change
Watford (F1)	3.6	2.0	-1.6
Holyhead (F.7)	3.5	2.2	-1.4
Sutton (NF)	3.8	3.1	-0.7
Gwalchmai (F1)	3.2	2.9	-0.3
Bodafon (PF)	3.2	3.6	+0.4

Another British study, carried out in Kilmarnok, Scotland, examined the tooth decay rates of permanent teeth (DMFT) of 9- to 14-year-olds. From the results, tabulated below, it is hard to discern any significant beneficial effect from fluoride.

EFFECT OF FLUORIDE ON TOOTH DECAY RATES IN HUMANS

Age	9	10	11	12	13	14
DMFT 1956	3.4	4.4	5.8	7.4	9.1	9.0
DMFT 1968	3.7	4.1	4.9	6.6	8.4	9.6
Change from 1956 to 1968	+0.3	-0.3	-0.9	-0.8	-0.7	+0.6
No. of Years Fluoride was Consumed	3	4	5	6	6.5	6.5

Recent Large-Scale Studies Show Fluoridation Does Not Reduce Tooth Decay in Permanent Teeth

Virtually every recent large-scale study done has shown that fluoridation does not reduce tooth decay in permanent teeth.

Dr. John Colquhoun, former Chief Dental Officer of the Department of Health in Auckland, New Zealand, examined the tooth decay rates of all 12- to 13-year-old students undergoing their final dental examination by the New Zealand Dental Service in 1984 and 1986 in the six major cities of New Zealand. This study included 59,331 students, the largest study ever done in the world. As can be seen in the following table, no difference in tooth decay rate of permanent teeth was observed as a result of fluoridation.

TOOTH DECAY RATES (THE NUMBER OF DECAYED, MISSING & FILLED PERMANENT PER CHILD) AMONG 12- TO 13-YEAR-OLDS IN NEW ZEALAND

City	Fluoridation Status	Number of Students Examined	Decayed, Missing & Filled Permanent Teeth Per Child
Christchurch	Nonfluoridated	14166	3.05
Hamilton	Fluoridated	8065	3.20
Dunedin	Fluoridated	3955	2.90
Palmerstown North	Fluoridated	3771	3.15
Greater Auckland	Fluoridated	39404	2.95
Wellington	Fluoridated	17368	2.80

In the largest study of fluoridation and tooth decay ever done in the history of the United States, Dr. Yiamouyiannis examined data from the dental examinations (performed under contract from the United States Public Health Service in 1986-1987) of 39,207 schoolchildren, aged 5-17, in 84 areas throughout the United States. Of these areas, 27 had been fluoridated for 17 years or more (F), 30 had never been fluoridated (NF), and 27 had been only partially fluoridated or fluoridated for less than 17 years (PF). The average number of decayed, filled, and missing teeth per child (DMFT) were 1.96 in the F areas, 2.18 in the PF areas, and 1.99 in the NF areas. For life-long residents these values were 1.97 in the F areas, 2.25 in the PF areas, and 2.06 in the NF areas. In neither case was there any difference in tooth decay rate that could be attributed to fluoridation.

And there was no difference in the decay rate of permanent teeth in fluoridated and nonfluoridated areas at any age, as can be seen in the following figure.

TOOTH DECAY IN FLUORIDATED (F), PARTIALLY
FLUORIDATED (PF), AND NONFLUORIDATED (NF) AREAS:
PERMANENT TEETH

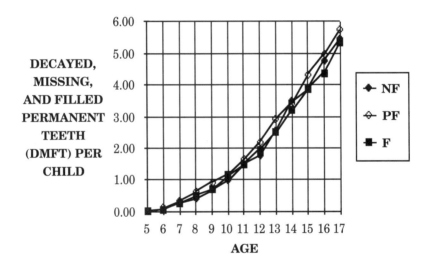

And the following table shows that when the 84 areas examined are put in the order of increasing decay rates of permanent teeth and compared, no dental benefit can be found as a result of living in a fluoridated area.

TOOTH DECAY RATES FOR 5- TO 17-YEAR-OLDS IN THE
U.S. IN THE ORDER OF INCREASING AGE-ADJUSTED
DMFT RATE (DECAYED, MISSING, AND FILLED
PERMANENT TEETH PER CHILD).

City	Fluoridation Status	Number of Students Examined	DMFT Per Child
Buhler, KS	Nonfluoridated	543	1.23
El Paso, TX	Fluoridated	451	1.32
Brooklyn, CT	Nonfluoridated	410	1.42
Richmond, VA	Fluoridated	475	1.44
Ft. Scott, KS	Fluoridated	491	1.44
Prince George, MD	Fluoridated	443	1.49
Cloverdale, OR	Nonfluoridated	354	1.49
Alliance, OH	Part. Fluoridated	467	1.58
Martin Co., FL	Nonfluoridated	440	1.59
Andrews, TX	Fluoridated	455	1.59
Coldspring, TX	Nonfluoridated	406	1.59
Tulsa, OK	Fluoridated	504	1.60
Palm Beach, FL	Nonfluoridated	476	1.61
Holcumb, MO	Part. Fluoridated	558	1.63
Kitsap, WA	Nonfluoridated	564	1.64
St. Louis, MO	Fluoridated	491	1.64
Houston, TX	Part. Fluoridated	488	1.66
Clarksville, IN	Fluoridated	428	1.68
Grand Island, NE	Nonfluoridated	535	1.72
Ft. Stockton, TX	Fluoridated	415	1.72
San Antonio, TX	Nonfluoridated	422	1.74
Cherry Creek, CO	Fluoridated	441	1.76
Tuscaloosa, AL	Fluoridated	475	1.81
Marion Co., FL	Part. Fluoridated	545	1.82
Cleveland, OH	Fluoridated	486	1.82
Allegany, MD	Nonfluoridated	458	1.83
Norwood, MA	Part. Fluoridated	434	1.84
Alton, IL	Fluoridated	511	1.86
Shamokin, PA	Nonfluoridated	462	1.86
Lodi, CA	Nonfluoridated	573	1.88
Bullock Creek, MI	Part. Fluoridated	472	1.88

Marlboro, MA	Part. Fluoridated	386	1.89
Allen, TX	Part. Fluoridated	445	1.91
San Francisco, CA	Fluoridated	456	1.91
E.Orange, NJ	Nonfluoridated	401	1.91
Lincoln/Sudbury, MA	Part. Fluoridated	436	1.92
Conejo, CA	Nonfluoridated	620	1.93
Lakewood, NJ	Nonfluoridated	450	1.93
New York City, NY-2	Fluoridated	336	1.95
Bethel, WA	Part. Fluoridated	540	1.96
Beach Park, IL	Fluoridated	518	1.97
Rising Star, TX	Part. Fluoridated	370	1.97
Philipsburg, PA	Fluoridated	499	1.98
Lanett, AL	Fluoridated	503	1.99
Plainville, CT	Part. Fluoridated	436	2.01
Wichita, KS	Nonfluoridated	496	2.04
Newark, NJ	Nonfluoridated	494	2.04
Knox Co., TN	Part. Fluoridated	530	2.06
Los Angeles, CA	Nonfluoridated	540	2.06
Pittsburgh, PA	Fluoridated	415	2.06
Lincoln, NE	Part. Fluoridated	476	2.08
Newton, KS	Nonfluoridated	464	2.08
Lakeshore, MI	Part. Fluoridated	486	2.09
New Paltz, NY	Nonfluoridated	350	2.11
Bemidgi, MN	Fluoridated	485	2.12
Alpine, OR	Nonfluoridated	397	2.13
Canon City, CO	Nonfluoridated	463	2.16
Wyandank, NY	Nonfluoridated	396	2.16
Millbrook, NY	Nonfluoridated	332	2.18
Chowchilla, CA	Nonfluoridated	551	2.18
New York City, NY-1	Fluoridated	503	2.19
Baltic, SD	Part. Fluoridated	487	2.19
Blue Hill, NE	Part. Fluoridated	480	2.22
Crawford, PA	Nonfluoridated	492	2.22
New Orleans, LA	Part. Fluoridated	459	2.25
Memphis, TN	Part. Fluoridated	464	2.25
Madison Co., MS	Part. Fluoridated	493	2.26
Milwaukee, WI	Fluoridated	478	2.35
Tooele, UT	Nonfluoridated	519	2.37
Chicopee, MA	Nonfluoridated	453	2.39

Cambria, PA	Part. Fluoridated	532	2.46
Springfield, VT	Part. Fluoridated	444	2.49
Dearborn, MI	Fluoridated	491	2.50
Maryville, TN	Fluoridated	466	2.51
Taunton, MA	Part. Fluoridated	445	2.52
Greenville, MI	Fluoridated	556	2.56
Hart/Pentwater, MI	Part. Fluoridated	455	2.58
Philadelphia, PA	Fluoridated	463	2.65
Sup. Union#47, VT	Part. Fluoridated	487	2.71
Cutler/Orosi, CA	Nonfluoridated	528	2.80
Brown City, MI	Fluoridated	512	2.97
Lawrence, MA	Part. Fluoridated	339	3.01
State of Hawaii	Nonfluoridated	293	3.29
Concordia Co., LA	Part. Fluoridated	424	3.77

The results in this study are comparable to those obtained in other large studies conducted in North America.

In 1989, researchers from Missouri examined the tooth decay records of rural 6th grade schoolchildren and again found no significant difference in tooth decay rates between those living in fluoridated areas (who averaged 2.2 decayed, missing, and filled teeth per child) and those living in nonfluoridated areas (who averaged 2.0 decayed, missing, and filled teeth per child).

The October, 1987 issue of the ***Journal of the Canadian Dental Association*** published an article admitting that fluoridation isn't doing the job that dentists have been claiming it could do. According to the article: *"Survey results in British Columbia with only 11% of the population using fluoridated water show lower DMFT rates than provinces with 40-70 per cent of the population drinking fluoridated water"* and *"school districts recently reporting the highest caries-free rates in the province were totally unfluoridated."*

Trends

Many studies show that in the United States and worldwide, reductions in tooth decay rates over the last 25 years in nonfluoridated areas and fluoridated areas have been comparable. People who extol the benefits of fluoride seem to ignore this fact.

Between 1958 and 1978, Dr. Robert Glass, a researcher at the Forsyth Dental Center in Boston, derived what he called 'amazing' statistics from a study of tooth decay in two nonfluoridated Boston suburbs, Norwood and Dedham. For the study, he examined the teeth of 1,776 children in the school systems of these two communities and discovered, over the course of 20 years, a 50 percent drop in the number of decayed, filled, and missing teeth.

Other studies from the United States as well as Australia, New Zealand and Britain, have also reported a 50 percent decrease in tooth decay in nonfluoridated areas.

Fluoridation Reduces Tooth Decay in Baby Teeth

In 1990, Dr. Yiamouyiannis carefully focused in on the number of decayed and filled baby teeth (dft) in children 5-8 years old who were permanent residents of fluoridated and nonfluoridated areas. Among 5-year-olds, he found that the decay rates of baby teeth in fluoridated areas were 42% lower than in the nonfluoridated areas, and that the difference was statistically significant. However, this reduction soon disappeared as children grew older, as can be seen from the following table.

PERCENTAGE REDUCTION IN dft RATES
IN LIFE-LONG RESIDENTS OF FLUORIDATED AREAS
IN COMPARISON TO NONFLUORIDATED AREAS

Age	Percent Reduction	Statistically Significant?
5	42%	Yes
6	18%	No
7	11%	No
8	1%	No

Fluoride may have caused this reduction in dft — simply by delaying baby tooth eruption. Recent studies examining 5-year-olds have indicated delayed eruption as a result of fluoridation that could account for such a difference in tooth decay rates. Delaying the eruption of baby teeth gives them less time to decay.

Decay-Free Children in Fluoridated and Nonfluoridated Areas

The percentage of children with no tooth decay in nonfluoridated areas is as high as or higher than it is in fluoridated areas, as can be seen from the following table.

PERCENTAGE OF DECAY-FREE CHILDREN IN FLUORIDATED AND NONFLUORIDATED AREAS

	Fluoridation Status	Number of Students Examined	Percent of Decay-free Children
5- to 17-year-olds 1986-1987			
United States	Nonfluoridated	13,882	35%
United States	Fluoridated	12,747	35%
12- to 13-year-olds 1984 and 1986			
Christchurch	Nonfluoridated	14,166	24%
Hamilton	Fluoridated	8,065	19%
Dunedin	Fluoridated	3,955	21%
Palmerstown North	Fluoridated	3,771	20%
Greater Auckland	Fluoridated	39,404	23%
Wellington	Fluoridated	17,368	24%

Good Diet, Not Fluoride, Necessary for Healthy Teeth

In primitive societies whose drinking waters contain negligible amounts of fluoride, such as the Otomi Indians in Mexico, the Bedouins in Israel, and the Ibos in Nigeria, 80 to 90 percent of the people go through life without tooth decay — not because the fluoride level in the drinking water is low, but because they eat very little sugar and other refined carbohydrates. More recent studies show that people living in low-fluoride areas who eat low-sugar diets experience very little tooth decay, whether they are 12-year-old schoolchildren in Tanzania or 20- to 50-year-old soldiers from Indonesia.

Fluoride in Toothpastes, Mouthrinses, Tablets, Drops, etc.

The only form in which fluoride may be effective in reducing tooth decay is the fluoride found in toothpaste. Children living on a high-sugar cariogenic diet who conscientiously brush their teeth may experience a 10% reduction in tooth decay as a result of the fluoride found in their toothpaste. But even here there is controversy, with some researchers claiming that fluoride toothpastes don't reduce tooth decay at all — and others claiming that higher levels of fluoride are needed to make toothpastes more effective — and still others claiming that lower levels are either as effective or more effective. Considering the hazards and potential gum-damaging effects of fluoride toothpastes (see Chapter 2), it would be best to keep fluoridated toothpastes out of the house.

Other forms of fluoride create a serious threat to health with no real benefit. Like water fluoridation, the apparent 'beneficial' effect of fluoride tablets is to retard the decay rates of baby teeth in 5- and 6-year-olds. Balance that against chronically poisoning your child, and very possibly leaving the tell-tale evidence of that poisoning in the form of dental fluorosis of the permanent teeth.

Chapter 15

See How They Pollute

"The garbage truck has to stop somewhere."
John Yiamouyiannis, 1983

"In regard to the use of fluosilicic acid as a source of fluoride for fluoridation, this agency regards such use as an ideal environmental solution to a long-standing problem. By recovering byproduct fluosilicic acid from fertilizer manufacturing, water and air pollution are minimized, and water utilities have a low-cost source of fluoride available to them."
Rebecca Hammer
Deputy Assistant Administrator
U.S. Environmental Protection Agency
March 30, 1983

If fluoridation creates such a public health hazard and does not significantly reduce tooth decay, why was fluoride ever added to the water supply? How is it that many areas around the country are still adding fluoride to the water supply?

Fluoride is an industrial waste product. The 1920s and 1930s saw the astronomical growth of the aluminum and phosphate fertilizer industries. Their growth gave rise to severe pollution problems. The pollutant—fluoride.

Fluoride pollution of air damaged wildlife, crops, and livestock. Initially, these industries bought up the surrounding fluoride-devastated areas. But when fluoride began to take its toll in human health, lawsuits and action by health officials forced the companies to install pollution-control devices to trap the fluoride waste products. Unfortunately, this just shifted the problem from airborne fluorides to waterborne fluorides and solid fluoride waste products, which were left to pollute rivers, streams, and ground waters. One means of profitably disposing of fluoride was to sell it as a rat poison and insecticide. However, since there weren't enough rats and insects around to poison, there still remained a problem of what to do with this excess fluoride. In addition, since fluoride is not biodegradable, excessive use of it as an insecticide and rodenticide would soon create a health hazard for humans.

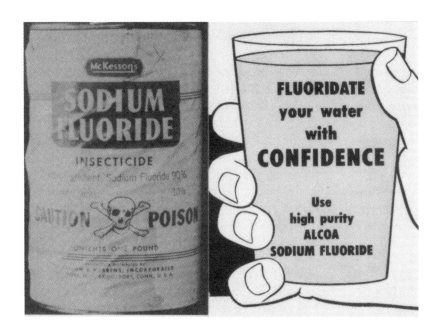

Dr. Gerald Cox of the Mellon Institute (the Mellons were owners of the Aluminum Company of America—ALCOA) solved this problem: Dump the waste fluoride into public drinking water. Tell the people it will reduce tooth decay.

Joined by the American Dental Association, the aluminum and fertilizer industries began to promote the sale of fluoride to public water systems as a means to reduce tooth decay. Due to extensive lobbying from the dental professional-fluoride industrial complex, the U.S. Public Health Service prematurely endorsed fluoridation.

Ralph Nader points out: *"With the Public Health Service, the fluoride companies and the dentists on one side, and the consum-*

ers on the other side — fluoridation has been promoted without giving consumers their free choice. The average dentist goes along because his dental society passed a resolution about fluoridation years ago." (Address at Muhlenberg College, 1974)

Despite the attempts of the U.S. Public Health Service and the fluoride-polluting companies and the American Dental Association to get rid of this toxic waste product by dumping it into the public drinking water, the expense of removing sufficient fluoride from the emissions of fluoride polluters is too great and fluoride pollution around these factories continues. Aluminum and phosphate fertilizer manufacturers from Bellingham, Washington to Polk County, Florida, continue to be a health hazard to citizens in surrounding areas (see Chapter 2).

The July 30, 1979 issue of **Maclean's** magazine relates the following story concerning fluoride from an aluminum plant in New York State polluting Cornwall Island, located in the St. Lawrence River.

"James Thompson pulls open the barbed wire gate leading to a grassy pasture and, with two mongrel dogs at his heels, steps inside to inspect his 50 head of Hereford cattle, all dying slowly from fluoride poisoning. His herd stands in miniature; stunted, only waist-high. Calves are sometimes stillborn. The cows, after four years, can't chew hay because their teeth, like chalk, have been ground down to the gums. 'As soon as they start getting skinny I sell them,' says Thompson. 'Otherwise, they just starve.' He points across the river to the Reynolds Metals Company, discharging 75 pounds of fluoride per hour into the air, and shakes his head. 'And I helped build that place,' he sighs."

Dr. Lennart Krook, Dean of Postgraduate Research at Cornell University, examined the cattle on Cornwall Island and published his findings in the April 1979 **Cornell Veterinarian** and reported:

"Chronic fluoride poisoning in Cornwall Island cattle was manifested clinically by stunted growth and dental fluorosis to a degree of severe interference with drinking and mastication. Cows died at or were slaughtered after the third pregnancy. The deterioration of cows did not allow further pregnancies."

Lawrence Francis, chief of the 1500 Mohawk Indians living on the island, warns of the dangers of living near aluminum smelters and tells residents of other areas where projects to build new smelters are planned:

"Block the project. Block them with everything you have. If you fail, then move. Move as quickly as you can . . . because there's no money that can buy your health back."

The August 7, 1977 issue of the **Washington Post** carried an extensive article on the damage being done to cattle in Maryland. The **Post** reports:

"In the last four years, herds within a two-mile radius of the [Eastalco aluminum] plant have been plagued with intermittent fever, fits of coughing, and lameness. On some farms, at least two or three cows have died of slow deterioration and starvation. The hooves of some cows are elongated and curved like grotesque elf shoes.

"The cows crawl on their knees when they go lame. A calf, born in Pat Zimmerman's barn last fall, crawled for three days desperate to stand and nurse. It died of exhaustion. Half the farmers involved complain that it is difficult to breed their animals. Six of Austin Putman's cows aborted just before they reached full term this spring.

"In recent months, members of all six farm families and at least a dozen of their non-farm neighbors have also noticed changes in their own health. They complain of dizzy spells, nausea, arthritic pains and muscle aches, burning eyes, sore throats and fatigue. Some develop small brown spots on their limbs."

The August 14, 1977 issue of the **Sarasota Herald-Tribune** reports:

"Manatee, Hillsborough and Polk counties suffer four times the fluoride air pollution burdens which apparently have caused acute fluorosis of cattle in Maryland. The impacts of the Florida pollution, however, have been carefully concealed by the phosphate companies from whose mills the pollutants belch.

"The cattle grazing the pastures polluted by the poisonous chemical are owned either by the phosphate companies or by cattlemen leasing the land from the companies.

*"According to several sources contacted by the **Herald-Tribune**, complaint of pollution by a cattleman is sufficient cause for termination of his lease.*

"As a result, diseased cattle rarely surface at the state's veterinary diagnostic clinic, are treated privately if at all and are seldom mentioned as clinical examples in recent professional literature on the medically unique diseases."

Fluoride-contaminated phosphate is shipped from these areas and used as a fertilizer, as a supplement in animal feed, and as an ingredient or additive in foods.

When fluoride is not adequately removed from phosphate used in foods and feeds, the results are disastrous.

For example, Drs. F. F. V. Atkinson from the National Biological Standards Laboratories in Canberra, Australia and Gordon C. Hard of the Department of Veterinary Pathology of the University of Sidney, Australia reported that fluoride-contaminated phosphate supplements used for animal feed wiped out a significant part of the guinea pig population in Australia. Drs. Atkinson and Hard pointed out:

"Deaths often reaching epidemic proportion occurred in at least 8 major guinea-pig breeding units in Sidney and Canberra during 1964 and early 1965. Affected animals were characterized by loss of weight, depression, and inappetence, a marked slobbering causing saturation and open excoriation [a raw irritated lesion] of the chin, neck and venter [abdomen], and ultimate death. All ages were affected, but newly-weaned animals and pregnant or post-parturient females [females which have just given birth] appeared especially susceptible. Decrease in weight was evident for 1 to several weeks until increasing loss of fluid from the oral cavity presaged death within 5-20 days."

The September 30, 1977 **Detroit Free Press** reported that Dr. Donald Hillman, a veterinarian at the Department of Dairy

Science at Michigan State University, found that many cattle deaths and illnesses that had been attributed to feed pollution by PBBs (polybrominated biphenyls) were actually caused by high fluoride contents in the feeds. Dr. Hillman reported his findings more fully in the *Journal of Dairy Science*. He found high levels of fluoride in these animals along with the reduced thyroid activity and disrupted immune function characteristic of fluoride poisoning.

The August 14, 1981 issue of the *Grand Rapids (Michigan) Press* reported that the state's Toxic Substance Control Commission warned that a series of mysterious dog ailments at kennels in Michigan may be the result of fluoride contamination of pet foods. They noticed a high incidence of deformed puppies and pointed out that chronic effects of fluoride poisoning may not be noticeable for a long time.

The aluminum and phosphate manufacturers, while responsible for the most intensive fluoride pollution, are not the only fluoride-polluting industries. Joining the aluminum and phosphate manufacturers in their fluoride-polluting activities are the steel, coal-burning power, clay, glass and non-ferrous metals industries.

On January 4, 1986, the nuclear industry added its name to the list of fluoride-polluting industries. James Harrison died and other workers at Kerr McGee were hospitalized when a nuclear fuels processing plant operated by Kerr McGee near Webber Falls, Oklahoma exploded, releasing over 14 tons of radioactive uranium hexafluoride. The uranium hexafluoride reacted with the moisture in the air to produce fluoride and a uranium residue. In reporting the story, the January 7, 1986 issue of the *San Jose [California] Mercury News* reported, *"Richard Cunningham, safety-division director at the Nuclear Regulatory Commission, said Monday that Harrison and five other workers also may have inhaled 'a small amount of uranium' but that their burns and respiratory distress were caused by the nonradioactive chemical [fluoride]."*

On October 30, 1987, a massive leak of hydrogen fluoride gas from a Marathon Oil plant in Texas City sent thousands fleeing and hundreds to the hospital. The October 31, 1987 issue of the *Houston Post* ran the headline *"4,000 flee Texas City acid spill, 223 hurt, 5-square-mile area evacuated after vapors spew into the air".* On November 20, 1987, the *Houston Post* reported that the *"Texas City acid leak could have rivaled Bhopal".* The November 22, 1987 *Houston Post* ran the headline *"Federal expert says Texas City was close to massive tragedy, Thousands could have been killed."* From the accounts of consumer activists in the area, all Marathon Oil did was try to minimize the tragedy and get their lawyers to settle claims 'for pennies' before the residents of the area could determine the severity of the harm done to them.

What would happen if it was ever officially admitted that low levels of fluoride are hazardous to human health? The consequences to industry in terms of lawsuits and pollution-control costs would be enormous. Is it surprising, then, that ever since the 1930s, industry and government have claimed that fluoride is safe and good for you?

Chapter 16

The Conspiracy: Early History

*"Perhaps the greatest deterrent to meaningful political engage-
ment of dentists in the promotion of water fluoridation is the
mistaken but widespread assumption that to do so they must
have full and complete knowledge of the detailed and voluminous
scientific literature on the relationship of water fluoridation to
dental and general health. They do not. . . . as soon as dentists
recognize their responsibility in the politics of fluoridation, their
performance will be outstanding. In politics, the emphasis is on
propagandizing rather than education."*
British Dental Journal
September 15, 1970, page 300

At the turn of the century, damage to teeth was observed in
various areas which by 1931 was found to be due to fluoride in
the water (see Chapter 5). This finding resulted in the American
Dental Association (ADA) and the U.S. Public Health Service
(USPHS) calling for the removal of fluoride from waters where it
naturally occurred and from the air where it was found as a
result of industrial contamination.

Court actions were filed against the polluters for personal
injury and these industries were also restricted from using the
water for the disposal of their waste fluorides.

In the 1930s, H. Trendley Dean of the USPHS conducted
extensive surveys showing that, as fluoride levels in the water
increased, so did this characteristic damage to the teeth, now
referred to as dental fluorosis. Then Dr. Gerald Cox, who was on
the staff of the Mellon Institute (the Mellons were the owners of
ALCOA Aluminum), got involved, claiming that if some fluoride
was bad for the teeth, a smaller amount would be good for the

teeth. He suggested (without any evidence) that 1 ppm fluoride was the proper dose and that in areas where it was lower than 1 ppm, it should be added to the water supply. This provided a means for fluoride-polluting industries (aluminum and phosphate fertilizer plants) to use the drinking water as a sewer for their toxic fluoride waste products. and to convince health officials to soften restrictions on the use of rivers and streams for dumping fluoride.

In the late 1930s, Dean started publishing purposely skewed data to show that, at 1 ppm, fluoride produced a minimal amount of dental fluorosis and resulted in the reduction of tooth decay (see Chapter 14). In 1931, when Dean's studies were initiated under the sponsorship of the USPHS, the USPHS was under the jurisdiction of Treasury Secretary Andrew Mellon (founder of ALCOA aluminum), who expressed his personal 'interest' in studies of fluoride's effects on humans.

Despite the ALCOA-dominated 1-2 punch of Dean and Cox, there were two major obstacles in the campaign to promote fluoridation: the American Medical Association and the American Dental Association. As late as September 18, 1943, the ***Journal of the American Medical Association*** pointed out:

"Distribution of the element fluoride is so widespread throughout nature that a small intake of the element is practically unavoidable. Fluorides are general protoplasmic poisons, probably changing the permeability of the cell membrane by inhibiting certain enzyme systems. The exact mechanism of such actions is obscure. The sources of fluorine intoxication are drinking water containing 1 part per million or more of fluorine, fluorine compounds used as insecticidal sprays for fruits and vegetables (cryolite and barium fluosilicate) and the mining and conversion of phosphate rock to superphosphate, which is used as fertilizer. The fluorine content of phosphate rock is about 4 percent. During conversion to superphosphate, about 25 percent of the fluorine present is volatilized and represents a pouring into the atmosphere of approximately 25,000 tons of pure fluorine annually. Another source of fluorine intoxication is from the fluorides used in the smelting of many metals, such as steel and aluminum, and in the production of glass, enamel and brick."

The October 1, 1944 issue of the *Journal of the American Dental Association* warned that:

"We do know the use of drinking water containing as little as 1.2 to 3.0 parts per million of fluorine will cause such developmental disturbances in bones as osteosclerosis, spondylosis and osteopetrosis, as well as goiter, and we cannot afford to run the risk of producing such serious systemic disturbances in applying what is at present a doubtful procedure intended to prevent development of dental disfigurements among children.

"Because of our anxiety to find some therapeutic procedure that will promote mass prevention of caries, the seeming potentialities of fluorine appear speculatively attractive, but, in the light of our present knowledge or lack of knowledge of the chemistry of the subject, the potentialities for harm far outweigh those for good."

Despite these warnings, Dr. Cox had convinced a Wisconsin dentist, J.J. Frisch, to promote the addition of fluoride to the water supply. In his book, *The Fight for Fluoridation*, historian D.R. McNeil referred to Frisch as *"a man possessed. . . Fluoridation became practically a religion with him."* In his crusade, Frisch enlisted the support of Frank Bull who organized political campaigns in order to persuade local officials to approve fluoridation.

According to the May 25-27, 1954 *Hearings before the Committee on Interstate and Foreign Commerce*:

*"In 1944, Oscar Ewing was put on the payroll of the Aluminum Company of America, as attorney, at an annual salary of $750,000. This fact was established at a Senate hearing and became a part of the **Congressional Record**. Since the Aluminum Co. had no big litigation pending at that time, the question might logically be asked, why such a large fee? A few months thereafter, Mr. Ewing was made Federal Security Administrator with the announcement that he was taking a big salary cut to serve his country."*

The USPHS, then a division of the Federal Security Administration, was under Ewing's command, and began vigorously promoting fluoridation nationwide.

An article from the Fall 1992 issue of ***Covert Action*** fills in the next piece of the puzzle.

*"Oscar Ewing's public relation's strategist for the water fluoridation campaign was none other than Sigmund Freud's nephew Edward L. Bernays, 'The Original Spin Doctor', as a **Washington Post** headline recently termed him. Bernays, also known as the 'father of public relations,' pioneered the application of his uncle's theories to advertising and public propaganda. The government's fluoridation campaign was one of his most stunning and enduring successes.*

*"In his 1928 book **Propaganda**, Bernays explained 'the structure of the mechanism which controls the public mind, and how it is manipulated by the special pleader [i.e., public relations counsel] who seeks to create public acceptance for a particular idea or commodity . . . Those who manipulate this unseen mechanism of society constitute an invisible government which is the true ruling power of our country . . . our minds are molded, our tastes formed, our ideas suggested, largely by men we have never heard of . . .'*

"'If you can influence the [group] leaders,' wrote Bernays who had many confidential industrial clients, 'either with or without their conscious cooperation, you automatically influence the group which they sway. . .'

"Describing how, as PR man for the Beech-nut Bacon Company, he influenced leaders of the medical profession to promote sales, Bernays wrote, 'The new salesman [would] suggest to physicians to say publicly that it is wholesome to eat bacon. He knows as a mathematical certainty that large numbers of persons will follow the advice of their doctors because he understands the psychological relationship of dependence of men on their physicians.'

"Substitute 'dentists' for 'physicians' and 'fluoride' for 'bacon' and the similarities are apparent."

On July 24, 1944, the following announcement was made by City Manager Walter H. Sack to the members of the City Commission of Grand Rapids[3]:

---

[3] Record of the City Commission of Grand Rapids, July 24, 1944, p. 70.

"The State Department of Health is planning a long range experiment and have selected Grand Rapids as the city to use for it. In accordance with their request, I am asking you to meet with the Representatives from the University of Michigan, Federal Government and State Health Department . . . on Monday July 31."

On July 31, the City Commission of Grand Rapids approved a motion to fluoridate and on January 25, 1945, despite the warning issued three months earlier by the ADA, fluoride was added to the drinking water of Grand Rapids, Michigan, the first city in the U. S. to fluoridate its drinking water. It was to serve as the test city and its tooth decay rates were to be compared with those of nonfluoridated Muskegon, Michigan for ten years, at which time it would be determined whether or not fluoridation was safe and effective. Dr. H. Trendley Dean was put in charge of the project.

Covert Action continues: *"Almost overnight, under Bernays' mass mind-molding, the popular image of fluoride — which at the time was being widely sold as rat and bug poison — became that of a beneficial provider of gleaming smiles, absolutely safe, and good for children, bestowed by a benevolent paternal government. Its opponents were permanently engraved on the public mind as crackpots and right-wing loonies . . .*

"fluoridation made possible a master public relations stroke — one that could keep scientists and the public off fluoride's case for years to come. If the leaders of dentistry, medicine, and public health could be persuaded to endorse fluoride in the public's drinking water, proclaiming to the nation that there was a 'wide margin of safety,' how were they going to turn around later and say industry's fluoride pollution was dangerous?"

And they fell for it. In 1950, long before any studies had been completed to determine whether the addition of fluoride to the public water supplies was a safe and effective means for reducing tooth decay, the USPHS and the ADA endorsed fluoridation. Within a short time thereafter, Muskegon, the control city in the Grand Rapids study was fluoridated. These endorsements effectively overshadowed the fact that the tooth decay rate in nonfluoridated Muskegon had decreased about as much as in fluoridated Grand Rapids — and that fluoridation was ineffective in reducing decay in permanent teeth.

The USPHS formed an unholy alliance with the trade unions of medicine and industry to promote the addition of a toxic waste product to the public water supply, at a concentration already shown to damage teeth (mottling); its other health effects were as yet undetermined. As a result, these organizations put their reputations on the line to support a measure which would haunt them to its dying day.

In the following year, the USPHS, with the cooperation of the ADA, held a meeting of state dental directors at which the methods for promoting fluoridation were outlined. The main speaker at this 'pep rally', speaking under the title *"What Are We Waiting For?"* was Frank Bull, the director of dental education for the Wisconsin State Board of Health. With regard to the scientific facts of fluoridation, Dr. Bull stated: *"I hope we are right."*

His presentation dealt primarily with how to get fluoridation implemented and how to discredit and handle opponents of fluoridation by means of rhetorical trickery. Concerning dental fluorosis, he suggested the following:

"Now, we tell them this, that at one part per million dental fluorosis brings about the most beautiful looking teeth any anyone ever had. And we show them some pictures of such teeth. We don't try to say that there is no such thing as fluorosis, even at 1.2 parts per million, which we are recommending. But you have got to have an answer. Maybe you have a better one."

Dr. Bull suggested: *"Now in regard to toxicity — I noticed that Dr. Bain used the term adding sodium fluoride. We never do that. That is rat poison. You add fluorides. Never mind that sodium fluoride business . . . The question of toxicity . . . lay off it altogether. Just pass it over, 'We know there is absolutely no effect other than reducing tooth decay,' you say and go on."*

With regard to cancer, Dr. Bull commented: *"When this thing came out we never mentioned it in Wisconsin. All we did*

*was to get some publicity on the fact [sic] that there is less cancer
and less polio in high-fluoride areas. We got that kind of information out to the public so that if the opposition did bring up this
rumor they would be on the defensive rather than have us on the
defensive.*

*"The best technique is the reverse technique, not to refute the
thing but to show where the opposite is true."*

In 1952, the ADA, through a series of small 'pep talk' articles
written by Dr. Bull and his friends and published in the ***Journal of the American Dental Association***, instructed its
dentists:

*"In this matter of fluoridation it is not sufficient for a practic-
ing dentist to 'damn with faint praise' when a patient wishes to
discuss the process. He should not pass on to the patient his
personal opinions or hastily formed impressions but should use
the facts which are readily available to him. By so doing he will
be able to take the lead in preventing misunderstanding and
confusion and also be instrumental in bringing to his community
one of the best procedures yet discovered for control of dental
caries."*

In 1952, Dr. A.L. Miller, a United States representative from
Nebraska and Chairman of the Special Committee on Chemicals
in Foods, stated:

*"I am a former state health director and have always sup-
ported the Public Health Service in the measures that they
advocated. I am sorely disappointed that they now are advocat-
ing every single soul in the community should take fluoride
before all of the facts of experiments now in progress have been
completed.*

*"Mr. Speaker, it is disturbing to me when the men in the
Public Health Service, who, as late as 1950, were not ready to
endorse the universal use of fluorine, have now, almost to a man,
come out for the endorsement.*

*"It is difficult for me to understand how high officials in the
Public Health Service could change their mind, over a 3-month
period and completely reverse the field. Where once they advocated the go-slow sign on the use of fluorides they now apparently*

have gone overboard, and put out large amounts of propaganda favoring the fluoridation of water. I am certain that the dental profession merely echoes and endorses the opinions of the Public Health Service. They have done little experimental work themselves.

"Mr. Speaker, despite my best efforts, and from the evidence before my committee, I cannot find any public evidence that gave me the impression that the American Medical Association, the American Dental Association, or several other health agencies, now recommending the fluoridation of water, had done any original work of their own. These groups were simply endorsing each other's opinions.

"You will note that all of the experts grounded in the science of biochemistry have advocated the go-slow sign on the use of fluorides in drinking water. I believe that the dental profession and other public-minded individuals, like myself, have been misled by the Public Health Service, because all of the facts have not been made available upon this subject.

"One dentist even wrote me that dental caries might be the cause of poliomyelitis, and because I objected to the use of fluorine for everyone, I might be the cause of numerous cases of polio. How ridiculous that statement is from a man who should be a thinking scientific man.

"I sometimes wonder if the Aluminum Co. of America, and its many subsidiary companies might not have a deep interest in getting rid of the waste products from the manufacture of aluminum, because these products contain a large amount of fluoride. In this connection it is interesting to know that Oscar Ewing, who now heads up the Federal Security Administration [at that time the parent organization of the U.S. Public Health Service], and the firm of attorneys he deals with — Hubbard, Hill and Ewin — represents the Aluminum Co. of America."

In a few years, Procter and Gamble (P&G) got involved with the fluoride issue and the ADA by getting ADA's endorsement for its fluoridated toothpaste. As evidence mounted showing that fluoridation was unsafe and ineffective, scientists who came out with negative findings regarding fluoride and fluoridation were personally denigrated by the ADA and by the USPHS; the

research of those opposing fluoridation, often far better and
more rigorous than the research claiming that fluoridation was
safe and effective, was portrayed as being faulty or irrelevant.
Some of those opposing fluoridation were dentists: they were
censured or lost their membership to the ADA[4]. Those with
USPHS grants lost them or lost the chance of getting them[5].
Public health officials who spoke out lost their jobs[6]; others who
didn't speak out kept quiet for fear of losing their jobs.[7]

And the most ruthless liars took the lead engaging in a conspiracy to defraud the public claiming that fluoridation was
absolutely safe and effective when they knew it was not. A
strong, well-financed network evolved supported by the USPHS,
ADA, their state and local affiliates, and P&G. They were also
quietly supported by companies using our drinking water as a
sewer for their poisonous waste product.

Since the time that the promotion of fluoridation began,
scientific evidence has progressed to the point where it can be
shown that fluoridation is ineffective and responsible for the
chronic poisoning of over 130,000,000 Americans. To save their
reputations, the promoters of fluoridation have intimidated,
slandered, and lied. They have corrupted the legislative, judicial,
and administrative bodies of our government. They have even
perverted the very principles of science itself in their attempt to
cover up the damage they have done by promoting fluoridation.

---

[4] Dr. Max Ginns, see the Boston Daily Record, September 28, 1961.
[5] Dr. Aly Mohamed, Professor of Biology at the University of Missouri at
Kansas City.
[6] Dr. John Colquhoun, former Chief Dental Officer of Auckland, New Zealand.
[7] Dr. Brian Dimenti, former chief toxicologist of the Virginia Department of
Health.

Chapter 17

The Conspiracy:
The Second Generation

*"A bureaucrat is the most despicable of men, though he is needed
as vultures are needed, but one hardly admires vultures whom
bureaucrats so strangely resemble. I have yet to meet a bureaucrat who was not petty, dull, almost witless, crafty or stupid, an
oppressor or a thief, a holder of a little authority in which he
delights, as a boy delights in possessing a vicious dog. Who can
trust such creatures?"*

Cicero, circa 50 B.C.

At the center of the second-generation conspiracy is John
Small. While he is only a high school graduate with no college
degree, his credentials do include six years as an information
officer for a government department on chemical warfare. He is
now and has been the U.S. Public Health Service 'expert' on
fluoridation since the 1960s.

Mr. Small's functions at the USPHS include the writing and
printing of anonymous memos, on USPHS letterheads, covering
up the harmful effects of fluoridation, and distributing these
memos to promoters of fluoridation, and when necessary, getting his hands on memos and reports put out by the government
(even the White House[8]) and rewriting them so they no longer
express their original concerns about the toxicity and ineffective-
ness of fluoridation. Most of the information supplied to dentists

---

[8] In a letter, to Mike Easley and Colleen Wulf, John Small writes: "I thought
you should have a copy of the White House response to Y[iamouyiannis], in
case he excerpts, misinterprets, or otherwise abuses it. I also suggest that
this not be floated around or even mentioned unless there is a real need for a
specific response about it. T[hank]G[od] we got to see this — the early draft
was — well, you wouldn't have liked it. John (Small) 5-29-84.

and physicians concerning fluoridation comes either directly or indirectly from Mr. Small. He is the cover-up supervisor, an expert relied upon by the USPHS to supply answers to Congress.

He also has the task of harassing, intimidating, and destroying anyone whose publications, utterances, or activities work to the detriment of fluoridation. In some cases, he calls upon other divisions of the Public Health Service to 'neutralize' studies or articles showing adverse effects of fluoridation.

In 1969, when Dr. Yiamouyiannis was a biochemical editor for Chemical Abstracts Service, the world's largest chemical information center and the largest division of the American Chemical Society, he began to publicly express his concern about the health risks associated with fluoridation.

Mr. Small contacted his employer and communicated his displeasure with the statements of Dr. Yiamouyiannis. Dr. Yiamouyiannis was notified by his employer several times and finally told that if he spoke out against fluoridation one more time, he would be fired. He was told that $1.1 million in federal funding was in jeopardy if Chemical Abstracts Service did not shut him up.

After the meeting, his employer wrote to Small, *"I have again talked to Dr. Yiamouyiannis and I have again made my position as strong and as clear as possible. He will not repeat this kind of performance and remain as an employee of Chemical Abstracts Service."* Within weeks after Dr. Yiamouyiannis next spoke out against fluoridation, he was put on probation, was told that he would never receive a raise again, and was advised to find another job. He was ultimately forced to resign.

Two years later, Dr. Yiamouyiannis was appointed science director of the National Health Federation where he was able to devote more time on the fluoridation issue.

During the 1970s, the fluoridation battle was stalemated. On one side, those opposing fluoridation were winning elections to stop fluoridation. On the other side, there was the force and money and power of the USPHS, the ADA, and industry that kept fluoridation going. In 1978, Yiamouyiannis served as a consultant and witness in a court case in Pennsylvania that proved fluoridation was harmful and banned it. The fluoridation promoters had to do something.

ADA's White Paper

In 1979, the American Dental Association came out with a *"White Paper on Fluoridation"* characterizing fluoridation opponents as either *"uninformed or misinformed"* or *"self-styled experts whose qualifications for speaking out on such a scientific issue as fluoridation were practically nonexistent or whose motivation was self-serving"*. It suggested that dentists should propagandize politicians while they are in the dental chair. The White Paper proposed setting up the conspiracy between the American Dental Association, Centers for Disease Control, Environmental Protection Agency, National Center for Health Statistics, National Institute of Dental Research, state dental societies, and state dental directors for *"identification of communities where the timing for political action is favorable as well as unfavorable and where the opponents of fluoridation are considering the initiation of referendums"* and for *"promoting fluoridation"*.

It urged that *"individual dentists must be convinced that they need not be familiar with scientific reports . . . on fluoridation to be effective participants in the promotion program"* and that the ADA should cooperate with the USPHS to get EPA to soften its statements regarding fluoride as a contaminant. It suggested behavioral studies to *"help anticipate the behavior of opponents of fluoridation"*, e.g. studies that would determine *"Why would some persons deny the life-long health benefits of fluoridation to children? What kind of mentality would reject the opinion of those who are qualified by education, training and experience . . . "*.

It suggested that ADA's responses to opponents of fluoridation should be prefaced by: *"'The ADA reiterated its long-standing support of fluoridation . . . ', 'Numerous studies have shown . . . ', 'There is no evidence of any relation . . . ', 'Investigators have observed . . . '"*. It suggested that *"The advice of behavioral scientists should be sought with regard to more realistic, convincing rebuttals"* and that *"The ADA should produce a step-by-step manual for the development and conduct of a fluoridation campaign . . . The ADA should provide field assistance if needed in a fluoridation campaign or cooperate with the [US]PHS and state health departments in providing such assistance"*.

Strategies of the Second Generation

This conspiracy solidified in the formation of a planning commit-
tee to organize a symposium (sponsored by the United States
Department of Health and Human Services (USDHHS),
USPHS, Health Resources and Services Administration, Bureau
of Health Care and Assistance, Maternal and Child Health
Division, Centers for Disease Control, Center for Prevention
Services, Dental Disease Prevention Activity, the W. K. Kellogg
Foundation, Delta Dental Health Plan of Michigan, Blue Cross
and Blue Shield of Michigan, and Medical Products Laboratories). This symposium took place at the University of Michigan
on August 9-10, 1983.[9]

Members of the planning committee included Mr. Small, Mr.
James Collins of the CDC, Dr. Stephen Corbin of the USPHS,
Dr. Robert Mecklenburg, Chief Dental Officer of the USPHS, Dr.
William Warren, Chief Dental Officer of the Department of
Health and Human Services, Dr. Joel Boriskin[10], chairman of
the American Dental Association's National Fluoridation Advi-
sory Committee, Dr. Wilbert Fletke of the ADA, Dr. Anthony
Kiser of the ADA, Ms. M. Lisa Watson of the ADA, Ms. Martha
Liggett of the American Association of Dental Schools, Dr.
Michael Easley, formerly of the Ohio Dept. of Health and CDC,
and Dr. Ray Kuthy[11] of the Illinois Department of Health, who
were and/or are some of the central figures in the conspiracy.

The stated purpose of the meeting was to *"discuss the status
of organized opposition to fluoridation; to analyze probable
motives influencing the antifluoride movement; to assess the need
for a national fluoridation strategy; to develop political and legal
strategies for the defense and promotion of fluoridation; and to
evaluate past legal and political profluoridation initiatives,
focusing on the defeats as well as the victories."*

---

[9] The proceedings of the symposium were published in a 129-page book titled
"Fluoridation: Litigation and Changing Public Policy", edited by Michael Easley and
Coleen Wulf, Kerry J. Brayton, and David F. Stiffler.

[10] According to the May 1990 *Journal of the American Dental Association*. In a
11/21/88 address before the Calgary Health Department, he claimed: that "1500
milligrams of fluoride per day [a lethal dose] . . . is prescribed to older people that
have progressive hearing loss".

[11] Ray Kuthy testified as a profluoridation witness in the Illinois court case to stop
fluoridation and posed for pictures in "Yiamouyiannis sucks" T-shirts after losing the case.

An examination of the seminar speakers, their affiliation, and the content of their presentations provides a further look into the 'unamerican' nature of this taxpayer-supported event.

Speakers included:

Dr. William T. Jarvis, a member of the board of advisors of the American Council of Science and Health (ACSH)[12] and the National Council Against Health Fraud (NCAHF). He spoke on the *"Psychology of Antifluoridationism"*. With regard to those opposing fluoridation, he stated: *"I do not believe in providing such people a public platform from which they can create confusion and doubt about fluoridation . . . For several years I have put on fluoridation debates in my dental classes, taking surveys before and after to determine attitudes toward fluoridation. Invariably, each class became more antifluoridationist as a result of the debate."*

Dr. Sheldon Rovin[13], a member of ACSH and coauthor with Stephen Barrett of the book, **The Tooth Robbers,** a book defaming antifluoridationsits. He spoke on how to win fluoridation battles through the political process, pointing out that *"if it is at all humanly possible, the referendum should be avoided."* In the discussion following, Dr. Myron Allukian asked what could be done to stop antifluoridationists from getting signatures to put fluoridation on the ballot.

Dr. Stephen Corbin of the USPHS. As chairman of his workshop, he reported that his committee felt *"the lead entities, namely the U.S. Public Health Service and the American Dental Association"* should accept a plan *"to close the 'windows of vulnerability' in our defense"*. He suggested avoiding trials based on the merits of fluoridation. Finally, he suggested that a mandatory state fluoridation law be developed. During the following discussion, Dr. Easley suggested a conspiracy to deny those seeking relief through the courts their right to due process.

---

[12] a front group for the junk food industry, the chemical industry, and other polluters
[13] He made the following statement in **Journal of Public Health Dentistry**: "There are increasing numbers of 'credentialed opponents' lurking about in fluoridation matters . . . ignore them, assail their motivations, or drown them out by enlisting large numbers of dentists and physicians."

Dr. Dennis H. Leverett[14] of the University of Rochester. As chairman of his workshop, he reported that his committee felt that fluoridation was "*a political rather than a scientific situation*" and encouraged research on the adverse effects of fluoridation "*that will presumably show no effect or will show equivocal results*".

Dr. D. Scott Navarro of Blue Cross/Blue Shield, as chairman of his workshop, suggested that the cost of litigation defending fluoridation should be borne by taxpayers, professional organizations, health groups, universities, and research institutes.

Colleen Wulf of the Ohio Department of Health. As chairman of her workshop, she reported that her committee suggested the formation of a nonprofit organization which would coordinate with the CDC and ADA, pointing out that CDC has already drafted promotional materials for fluoride and that the ADA and the USPHS had already formed the Ad Hoc Committee to Plan for the Legal Defense of Community Water Fluoridation. She suggested that the name of the new group might be something like "'*Coalition for Improved Dental Health*' or something similar".

---

[14] In a letter to Dr. David Werdegar dated July 17, 1985 Leverett states "*I have raised some questions, particularly in a recent article in* **Science** *, Volume 217, pp. 26-30 (1982), which relate to current widely accepted norms for fluoride administration . . . I have never, even for an instant, believed that we are receiving too much fluoride . . . I argue only, in light of these facts, that we need to reassess our definition of 'optimal'. If I had to guess the outcome, I would say that we would be most likely to adjust the optimum dosage upward*". However, in the **Science** article quoted above, he makes himself out to be a liar. Under the section "Increasing Prevalence of Fluorosis", he states "*If there are increasing concentrations of fluoride in the food chain, particularly food for infants, then we would expect fluorosis to be increasing in the populations as well. This is, indeed, the case. . . In our own prevalence studies, we found mild fluorosis in 28 percent of children 11 to 13 years of age from communities with fluoridated water, whereas 12 percent would have been expected from Dean's studies . . . The widespread use of fluorides may have created a situation in which we are approaching a critical mass of fluoride in the environment . . . there needs to be extensive research addressing the issue of increased fluoride in the food chain . . . On the basis of the findings described in this article, the definition of the optimum concentration of fluoride in community water supplies needs to be reassessed.*"

ASLAP

As a matter of fact, the name of the group ended up being the American Oral Health Institute, incorporated in the state of Ohio on February 19, 1985 as a not-for-profit corporation. In 1985 and 1988, this organization came out with the first and second editions of a book, titled *Abuse of the Scientific Literature in an Antifluoridation Pamphlet* (ASLAP), edited by Coleen A. Wulf[15], Karen F. Hughes, Kathleen G. Smith[16], and Michael W. Easley. The 215-page second edition of this book attacked the 1982, 1983, 1986, and 1988 editions of a very well referenced Question and Answer pamphlet titled *Lifesavers Guide to Fluoridation* (LG) by Dr. Yiamouyiannis that was effectively being used to fight fluoridation.

The preparation of this book was a collaborative effort of 18 federal and state health officials who were promoting fluoridation. Those with an asterisk after their name were invited to or attended the University of Michigan on August 9-10, 1983 symposium discussed above. There was not a single scientist among them: 10 were dental hygienists (Colleen A. Wulf*, Karen F. Hughes*, Kathleen G. Smith*, Linda S. Crossett*, Elizabeth King, Sharon Pierce, Ruth Nowjak-Raymer, Beverly Wargo, Geraldine Wirthman, and Karen Zinner), 2 were dentists (Michael Easley* and Elizabeth Bernard), 5 had degrees in public relations, education, psychology, or public health (James Collins*, Taimi M. Carnahan*, Claire Gelband, Judy Harvey, and Helen S. Hill), and one had no college degree at all (John Small*). The person who wrote the introduction was a psychiatrist (Stephen Barrett*[17]).

---

[15] On February 4, 1983 she wrote a letter to her colleagues revealing some of the underpinnings of the conspiracy to produce ASLAP and implicating the CDC's Jim Collins and NIDR's John Small in its conception. In a subsequent meeting with Dr. Yiamouyiannis, she admitted that even if she were convinced that fluoridation were harmful, she would still continue promoting it.

[16] as Fluoridation Coordinator, PHS, Phoenix, AZ, she co-headed the profluoridation citizen group which asked the Phoenix Environmental Quality Commission to recommend the fluoridation of the Phoenix public water supply.

[17] see Chapter 19.

This lack of scientific expertise shows up in the text of ASLAP. On page 23, the ASLAP group refers to an article in which, they claim, female rats were exposed to hydroxyfluoride. However, the article they referred to makes no mention of hydroxyfluoride, since there is no such chemical. On pages 30 and 60, the ASLAP group tried to convert millimolar concentrations of fluoride into parts per million and were off in their calculations by 100,000%! On page 91, the ASLAP group was unable to determine what 'vitamin PP' was. Vitamin PP is niacinamide or vitamin B3.

Since science was not the area of expertise of the ASLAP group, what was? It appears that the ASLAP group substituted 'public relations' for science and truth in its attack on the LG.

In the introduction, they start off with an personal attack on Dr. Yiamouyiannis. Claims are then made that the references he used in the LG were out of date, were mostly not from reputable refereed scientific journals, did not support the claims attributed to them, are taken out of context, and are misrepresentations of legitimate scientific research. How do these charges stack up?

The references used in the LG were not out of date. The average date of publication of the references used in the 1988 LG was about 1975 and more than a third (over 70) of them were published in the 1980s. In contrast, the average date of publication of references used in the 1988 edition of ASLAP is about 1972-1973 and slightly less than a third of them were published in the 1980s.

Most of the references used in the LG are from refereed scientific journals. More than 70% of the references in the 1988 LG were original articles from refereed journals. By contrast, less than 25% of the references used by the 1988 edition of ASLAP group to support its case were original scientific articles from refereed journals.

Except for a few typographical and clerical errors, the references cited in the LG support the claims attributed to them. Of the 221 references cited in the LG, the ASLAP group take issue with only 29 of them. Of these 29 criticisms, 20 are without merit, 5 are judgement calls, and 4 are legitimate and are due to typographical and clerical errors.

Next, antifluoridationists in general and Dr. Yiamouyiannis in particular were declared to be guilty of *"deception"*, *"a marketing fraud"*, *"misrepresentations of scientific facts"*, of making *"fraudulent claims"*, of being responsible for *"the pain, suffering, nutritional compromise, economic loss, and social estrangement [of] . . . millions of American citizens"*, of using *"a pseudo-scientific approach"*, and of failing *"to demonstrate a fundamental knowledge of proper scientific documentation"*.

ADA and the EPA:
Their Involvement in the Fluoride Cover-Up

As a result of the passage of the Safe Drinking Water Act in 1974, U.S. Environmental Protection Agency rules were promulgated setting maximum contaminant levels, referred to as MCLs, for various water pollutants including fluoride. The MCL for fluoride was set at 1.4 parts per million for the warmer climates and at up to 2.4 parts per million for cooler climates. The ADA became concerned that by admitting harmful effects of fluoride were occurring at these low levels, the Environmental Protection Agency was interfering with ADA's political crusade to promote the addition of one part per million fluoride to the water supply.

Despite the fact that raising the MCL for fluoride would have devastating effects on children's teeth and on general health overall, the American Dental Association began pressuring the Environmental Protection Agency to raise the MCL to up to 8 parts per million. In their own publication, the American Dental Association admitted that its reasons for doing so was to keep its fluoridation crusade on track.

Centrally involved in the drive to raise the fluoride MCL were the ADA, ADA's Lisa Watson, John Small, Robert Mecklenberg, U.S. Chief Dental Officer, C. Everett Koop[18], U.S. Surgeon General, the USEPA crew of Joe Cotruvo, Michael B. Cook, Ken Bailey, Jack Ravan, Victor Kimm, Peter L. Cook, and Ed Ohanian, and ICAIR Life Systems, Inc.

---

[18] Koop did paid TV ads on taxpayers' time proclaiming that fluoridation was absolutely safe and that dental fluorosis is not an adverse health effect. He also did a profluoride video tape for the American Dental Association.

This took place under the United States Environmental Protection Agency administrations of Lee Thomas and William Ruckelshaus and has continued on since then.

The Environmental Protection Agency set up hearings to re-evaluate the MCL for fluoride. At these hearings, Lisa Watson, the spokesperson for the American Dental Association, was shown a slide of a child from an area with about 4 ppm fluoride occurring naturally in the drinking water. The dental fluorosis of the child's teeth was severe. More than half of some of the teeth had crumbled away as the result of dental fluorosis. When asked whether she thought this constituted an adverse health effect of fluoride, the ADA spokesperson replied *"No"*, claiming the crumbling away of over half of one's tooth is not a health problem but merely a cosmetic problem.

The USEPA's National Drinking Water Advisory Council didn't buy the American Dental Association's story, refused to recommend raising the MCL, and came close to recommending that it be lowered.

However, higher level bureaucrats in the USEPA, apparently already 'gotten to' by the ADA and, concerned that their own scientists would not prostitute themselves by producing a report justifying an increase in the MCL for fluoride, 'farmed out' the research work to a group called ICAIR Life Systems, Inc. from Cleveland, Ohio.

The USEPA contracted with ICAIR Life Systems, Inc. in Cleveland, Ohio to prepare their report which would pave the way for increasing the MCL for fluoride. Scientists in the USEPA refused to go along with the conspiracy's attempts to increase the MCL. Apparently, John Small chose the material to be reviewed by ICAIR and may have been instrumental in writing parts of the report itself. In particular, the recently prepared ASLAP report was uncritically incorporated into the USEPA report. The authors of the bogus report claimed:

1) Dental fluorosis is not observed below 2.0 parts per million — even though data cited by the draft report itself shows dental fluorosis at fluoride levels at 0.8 parts per million (see also Chapter 5).

2) "Dental fluorosis was not judged to be an adverse effect"

and *"teeth with fluorosis are desirable."* (see Chapter 5).

3) Skeletal fluorosis has not been found among people drinking less than 4 parts per million fluoride in their drinking water — when in fact as little as 0.7 to 2.5 parts per million has been shown to cause skeletal fluorosis (see Chapter 6).

4) Only one laboratory found that fluoride caused genetic damage — when in fact over ten laboratories did (see Chapter 8).

5) They could find *"no data concerning mutagenic effect of fluoride on humans"* — when in fact there are (see Chapter 8).

6) They could find *"no information on the teratogenicity of fluoride"* — when in fact there is (see Chapter 8).

7) They could find no information on the carcinogenicity of fluoride — when in fact there is (see Chapter 9).

8) The 1977 study of Yiamouyiannis and Burk showing a link between fluoridation and cancer did not take age, race, and sex into consideration — when, in fact, it did.

9) The 1977 study of Yiamouyiannis and Burk showing a link between fluoridation and cancer was criticized by three specific publications — when in fact not one of these even addressed the 1977 study.

The fraudulent nature of this report has recently been confirmed by a former ICAIR Life Systems employee, Dr. John Beaver, who worked on the 1991 follow-up to this report. He states: *"It was clear that they were selectively including the studies of certain authors and excluding the reports of others."* This misleading information was sent to the EPA who forwarded it on to the Subcommittee on Risk Assessment of Ingested Fluoride of the National Academy of Sciences for another 'independent' report.

EPA and the USPHS:
Their Involvement in the Fluoride Cover-Up

Meanwhile, the United States Environmental Protection Agency also asked the Surgeon General's office to review the literature on the health effects of fluoride in drinking water and to recommend safe levels. In response, the Surgeon General's office, which has endorsed fluoridation since 1950 and has been the world's major promoter of fluoridation, convened an ad hoc committee. This committee starred John Small and Robert Mecklenburg, who, at the same time, were involved in setting up the symposium discussed previously under the subheading 'Strategies of the Second Generation'. Costars included NIDR's James P. Carlos, and Joe Cotruvo and Ed Ohanian, responsible for the fluoride cover-up at the USEPA, along with other nationally known outspoken promoters of fluoridation.[19]

The Surgeon General's committee was well aware of ADA's pressure to get the MCL for fluoride raised to eight parts per million, as can be seen by committee member Dr. Stanley Wallach's comment, *"We are being asked to discuss the issue of allowing the levels to go up to eight"*. Mecklenberg continually insisted that teeth that were pitted and worn down as a result of severe dental fluorosis from fluoride in the water did not constitute an adverse health effect and urged the committee not to set an MCL so low that it would jeopardize fluoridation.

Dr. Stephen Marx followed this cue and during the meeting admitted:

> *"If we were just handling this as an environmental contaminant, we could say we begin to see fluorosis at two parts per million. So we want a safety factor of four. We recommend that it be kept below a half a part per million."*
>
> *"Clearly, we have to make an allowance here. We can't just talk about safety."*[20]

---

[19] other members included Stephen J. Marx, NIADDK, Akepati H. Reddi, NIDR, Karl Keller, NIEHS, Frank Smith, Univ. of Rochester, Herta Spencer, Heinz VA Hosp., Heinz, IL, Michael Kleerekoper, Henry Ford Hospital, Detroit, Robert Marcus, Palo Alto VA, Vincent Vigorretta, Hosp. for Special Surgery, NY, Bess Dawson Hughes, USDA Human Nutrition Research Center, Boston, MA, David Rowe, UCONN Health Center, and Stanley Wallach, VA Hosp., Albany NY; listed as consultants were C. Conrad Johnston, Indiana Univ. Sch. of Med., B. Lawrence Riggs, Mayo Clinic, and James Shupe, Utah State Univ. Listed as observers were Bill Lappenbusch, USEPA, Arnie Kuzmak, and Hugh Hanson.
[20] But that was exactly what this committee was asked to do — talk about safety without regard to any other claimed effect. This is how the Safe Drinking Water Act is written.

Dr. James Carlos stated:

"I would rather see no fluorosis. I would keep it at two".

Dr. Stanley Wallach concurred stating:

"You would have to have rocks in your head, in my opinion, to allow your child much more than two parts per million."

Dr. David Rowe concurred: *"I think we all agree on that."*

The vote was 10 to 2 that the maximum contaminant level of fluoride be set between 1.4 and 2.4 parts per million for children up to age nine.

Subsequently, however, the report was altered to recommend 4 parts per million as the MCL of fluoride. This change as well as others that softened the report were made without the knowledge of the committee members. Using this report and the fraudulent ICAIR Life Systems report, the USEPA increased the MCL of fluoride to 4 ppm.[21]

The Knox Report
The British Connection[22]

To further justify their decision, the USEPA also drew upon another report — the Knox report, published in 1985 and quickly and uncritically incorporated by them as a part of their report.

E. G. Knox was a likely person for the profluoridationists to have as chairman. In 1980, he had published a study based on an extremely limited survey without a control group which, he claimed, showed no evidence of a fluoride effect on congenital malformations. This report coincidentally came out at about the same time as a similar report with similar conclusions by CDC's Erickson.

The Knox report is little more than the argument of the profluoridationists in their defense of fluoridation in the court case of McColl vs. the Stathclyde Regional Council, including the same lies, obfuscations, and omissions with one exception. It did

[21] See also *Medical Tribune*, April 20 and 27, 1989.
[22] for more on the British connection, see Chapter 18.

make one important and significant correction of the results of Yiamouyiannis and Burk which corrected the increase in cancer death rate of the 45-64 year age group from 15 per 100,000 per year (reported in the first edition of this book) to about 8-9 per 100,000 per year (reported in the second and third editions of this book). Aside from this, none of the other calculations of Yiamouyiannis and Burk were substantively challenged. The remainder of the report is a waste of paper.

The report acknowledges *"We obtained additional information from the authors of some of the studies to assist with our assessments, and we are grateful for the help given."* All of those from whom this additional help was sought were authors of studies claiming fluoridation does not cause cancer and/or persons who testified in court that fluoride did not cause cancer.

Referring to *"The trials . . . in Grand Rapids and Newburgh"* the Knox report claimed that *"None of the reports indicated a risk of cancer from fluoride or fluoridation."* In fact, both of them did 'indicate' a risk of cancer from fluoride.

The report claimed that *"Kinlen, 1974 . . . reported no significant differences in cancer rates between high and low fluoride areas"*. During court testimony in 1978, Kinlen admitted that this same study showed that the cancer incidence at sites he felt would most likely be affected by fluoridation were 5% higher in the fluoridated areas he examined than in the nonfluoridated areas.

> Q. *"Doctor, did you go over those calculations as I had gone through them?"*
> A. *"Yes."*
> Q. *"Do they appear to be correct, sir?"*
> A. *"Yes."*
> Q. *"In other words, the figure for the fluoridated column appears to be 1.03, does it not?"*
> A. *"Yes."*
> Q. *"And the figure for the nonfluoridated area appears to be 0.98 does it not?"*
> A. *"Yes."*
> Q. *"And does that not indicate that the fluoridated group appeared to have approximately a five percent greater cancer incidence rate than the nonfluoridated group?"*

A. *"The left [the cancer incidence figure in the fluoridated column] was 5% larger than the right [the cancer incidence figure from the nonfluoridated column]"*.

The Knox Report criticizes the use of data from intercensal years[23] in the analyses of Yiamouyiannis and Burk saying *"It would be safer to avoid this source of possible error by adopting the normal practice of centering the calculation of the standardized mortality ratios (SMRs) on, or closely around, the census years, thus using population estimates which would be expected to be more reliable."* Confronted with such figures, i.e., figures taken on, or closely around, the census years, Sir Richard Doll, the leading profluoridation witness in the case of McColl vs. the Stathclyde Regional Council, admitted that there was an absolute increase in cancer death rate in fluoridated areas:

> Queen's Counsel. *"Well, the figures speak for themselves, don't they, and would you agree that in general terms they show, whichever method you use, that the fluoridated cities do worse than the nonfluoridated cities in comparison as to what happened between 1950 and 1970?"*
>
> Doll. *"Yes, I do agree, and that is why I said this paper was the first paper which I thought was of any consequence. . ."*

While the Knox report maintained that virtually all other studies except for those of Yiamouyiannis and Burk show no link between fluoridation and cancer, the following table lists a number of the studies that did show a link between fluoridation and cancer at the time the Knox report was prepared. In some of the following studies, errors and omissions in the original studies have been corrected:

---

[23] data from intercensal years uses populations estimated from drawing a straight line between populations determined by the census and are used routinely in epidemiological studies, including many of studies used in the Knox report to support its own conclusions.

OTHER STUDIES SHOWING A LINK
BETWEEN FLUORIDATION AND CANCER
AT THE TIME THE KNOX REPORT WAS PREPARED

Author	Year	Increase in Cancer Death Rate	Increase in Cancer Incidence
Austin	1975	40%	18%
Cecilioni	1977	15-25%	
Erickson	1978	4%	
Hagan	1954*	7%	
Heasman	1964*	8%**	
Hoover	1975		8-10%
Illinois Dept. of Health	1952*	8%	
Kinlen	1974***		5%
Knutson	1954	22%	
Mirisola	1964	4%	

*natural fluoridation   **gastric cancers   ***see Kinlen's testimony (above)

Chapter 18

The Conspiracy: 'Containing' the Cancer Link

In 1975, Dr. Yiamouyiannis published a preliminary survey showing that people in fluoridated areas had a higher cancer death rate than people in nonfluoridated areas. When this material got into the hands of Mr. Small, he enlisted the aid of Drs. Robert Hoover and Marvin Schneiderman of the National Cancer Institute to refute these findings. Dr. Hoover's first claim was that the nonfluoridated areas (Los Angeles and Houston) had relatively clean air and that the increase in cancer death rate in these areas was lower than in fluoridated areas because their lung cancer rates were lower. First, it is obvious that Los Angeles and Houston did not have clean air and secondly, Dr. Yiamouyiannis showed that the increase in cancer death rates in fluoridated areas was not due to lung cancer but to other cancers.

In 1975, Dr. Dean Burk, chief chemist of the National Cancer Institute (1939 to 1974), joined with Dr. Yiamouyiannis in performing additional studies which were published in the **Congressional Record** by Congressman James J. Delaney, author of the Delaney amendment prohibiting the addition of cancer-causing substances to food used for human consumption. Both of these reports confirmed the existence of a link between fluoridation and cancer.

In attempting to refute these findings, Dr. Hoover and Dr. Schneiderman claimed that Drs. Burk and Yiamouyiannis had not corrected their figures for age, race, and sex and that when such corrections were made, the increase in cancer death rate found by Burk and Yiamouyiannis disappeared.

In the fall of 1977, two full hearings on fluoridation and cancer were held before Representative L.H. Fountain's Congressional Subcommittee on Intergovernmental Relations. At these hearings, Dr. Yiamouyiannis showed that Dr. Robert

Hoover's group and Dr. Donald Taves of the University of Rochester, in adjusting for age, sex, and race, had left out 80 to 90% of the relevant data.

In addition, he pointed out that Dr. Hoover's group had made an error in its calculations. When these errors and omissions were corrected, the very same age-sex-race corrections used by Dr. Hoover and Dr. Taves, confirmed the results of Drs. Burk and Yiamouyiannis showing that approximately 10,000 excess cancer deaths per year could be attributed to fluoridation in the United States.

During the hearings, Congressman Fountain, chairman of the subcommittee, showed that Dr. Hoover and other National Cancer Institute officials had purposely withheld information from Drs. Burk and Yiamouyiannis and clandestinely sent erroneous data to Dr. Leo Kinlen and Sir Richard Doll, professors at Oxford University and representatives of the Royal College of Physicians, who published the erroneous data as if it were their own. Not content with this duplication of data, Dr. Kinlen passed the data on to Dr. David Newell and Peter Oldham, representatives of the Royal Statistical Society, who again republished the same erroneous data. As in the original Hoover study, when errors and omissions in these studies were corrected, they also confirmed the results of Drs. Burk and Yiamouyiannis showing that approximately 10,000 excess cancer deaths per year could be attributed to fluoridation in the United States.

(With the help of Congressman Fountain's staff, Dr. Yiamouyiannis was able to get the letters between Dr. Hoover and the British investigators, exposing the British Connection. These letters are reprinted in full in the appendix.)

Congress Asks for Animal Study on Fluoride and Cancer — the 'NTP Study'

At the conclusion of the hearings, after listening to testimony from both opponents and proponents of fluoridation, Congressman Fountain, chairman of the committee, stated that *"at the present time the carcinogenicity, or lack of carcinogenicity, of this substance is a question which remains unanswered"* and ordered the United States Public Health Service to conduct animal studies to see if fluoride causes cancer.

NCI's Dr. Herman Kraybill[24] was placed in charge of these studies. At the hearings, Kraybill stated: *"this will be the final study to confirm negativity of fluoride ion in carcinogenesis."* While he cited 13 studies which he claimed already showed no link between fluoridation and cancer, not one of them had anything to do with fluoridation and cancer. In a subsequent meeting with Dr. Yiamouyiannis, NCI Director Dr. Arthur Upton admitted that the studies cited by Kraybill had nothing to do with fluoride and cancer. During the same meeting, Upton agreed to have Yiamouyiannis serve on the protocol committee which was to design the NTP study. Yiamouyiannis was never consulted.

And the design and progress of the study was such a disaster that the first set of studies, performed from 1982 to 1984 had to be scrapped. The second set of studies were performed at Battelle Memorial Institute in Columbus, Ohio from 1985 to 1987. In 1988 to 1989, Battelle released their *"Narrative and Final Report"* to the NTP. The results were most disturbing because the study reported highly significant specific fluoride-related cancers (see Chapter 9). The NTP turned these data over to Experimental Pathology Laboratories who reclassified the diagnosis of every one of the rare liver cancers found in the fluoride-treated mice and deleted them from the data sheets. In addition, they deleted all diagnoses of metaplastic or precancerous cells found in the mouths of rats receiving fluoride in the drinking water. These altered data were subsequently sent on to the 'Pathology Working Group' on December 6-8, 1989.

On January 22, 1990, the National Toxicology Program issued a press release with data confirming findings of a link between fluoride and osteosarcomas as well as higher rates of oral cancers in rats. Within a week, the American Dental Association put out a press release stating that *"Water fluoridation remains the safest, most effective, and most economical public health measure to reduce tooth decay"*.

---

[24] In 1972, he had already been chosen to write a memo that fluoride doesn't cause cancer; on Aug. 8, 1982, the Houston Post reported the involvement of Kraybill and his boss, Richard H. Adamson in a cover up of the link between benzene and cancer with the cooperation of IARC which shortly put out a report that fluoride does not cause cancer.

On February 6, 1990, the National Institute of Environmental and Health Sciences released the National Toxicology Program pathology data tables with a cover letter by Dr. David G. Hoel claiming that *"there has not been any evidence that shows a relationship between fluoridation and cancer or other diseases in humans."* Hoel continued: *"Moreover, water fluoridation has proven highly effective in improving the nation's dental health by markedly reducing tooth decay."* He stated that until *"this department's . . . NTP staff . . . prepares a detailed analysis of the data . . . [and] outside scientists . . . review the data and the NTP analysis . . . the significance of the results cannot be determined"*. He claimed that until then, *"the many benefits of fluoride warrant continuation of the present policy designed to prevent tooth decay."*

Pathology Associates chaired the 'Pathology Working Group', whose members included three from the NTP staff, two from Experimental Pathology Laboratories, and one from Chemical Industry Institute of Technology (CIIT). Not a single member of the Battelle Memorial Institute was invited. However, listed among those participating in this group was an 'observer' from Procter and Gamble. In addition to agreeing to conceal the fact that rare liver cancers and oral precancerous cells were linked to fluoride in the drinking water, this group deleted one of the osteosarcomas out of the high fluoride treatment group, reducing the number from four to three and returned it to the NTP data unit which date-stamped it as being received on February 16, 1990. One member of the staff who was not in or associated with the organizations involved in deleting the fluoride-linked cancers, Dr. James Popp of CIIT, told Dr. William Hirzy of the EPA that the evidence is clear that fluoride is a carcinogen.

On March 30, 1990, NTP released the final edition of their report. In the NTP report's section on genetic toxicity, the study of Mohamed and Chandler, as well as the studies of many others showing that fluoride causes genetic damage, were omitted. Instead, studies such as those of Dr. George Martin[25] were relied upon heavily. In the NTP report's section on carcinogenicity, important studies showing that fluoride induces tumors and

---

[25] see Chapter 19 under the subheading "Death of Science"

cancers, promotes tumor growth rate, enhances the carcinogenicity of other chemicals, and increases human cancer rates,
which should have been covered in this section, were either
buried or ignored altogether. While leaving out most of the
important published studies regarding the carcinogenicity of
fluoride, the authors of the report had the audacity to acknowl-
edge *"an industry-sponsored [P&G] study as yet unreported"*.
Treatment of studies on fluoridation and human cancer were
similar to other reports cited above. Rather than reporting that
there was clear evidence that fluoride caused cancer, the NTP
claimed that the evidence was only equivocal.

On April 30, 1990, Kraybill, the person responsible for
designing the NTP study and now a consultant to American
Council of Science and Health (ACSH), came out at an ACSH
press conference explaining why the NTP study he designed was
no good. ACSH threatened to sue the EPA if it *"tries to undermine the public confidence in fluoride"*. As noted above, the
ACSH is riddled with key fluoride proponents.

Worried about the effect of the NTP's findings, the fluoridation promoters could use one of several strategies to get rid of
the fear that there was even a possible fluoride-cancer link.

A. They could have other research done to show that fluoride
does not cause cancer in animals.

B. They could have Robert Hoover and his friends at the
National Cancer Institute as well as others do studies to show
that fluoride doesn't cause bone cancer in humans.

C. They could apply another coat of whitewash to the NTP
report by having the U. S. Department of Health and Human
Services (USDHHS) come out with another report covering up
the harmful effects of fluoride.

In fact, they used all three strategies.

Strategy A

On March 5, 1990, the **ADA News** reported that P&G had
unpublished findings which refuted the carcinogenicity of
fluoride. Shortly thereafter, P&G published their paper on
fluoride and bone cancer in rats only, and left out their data on

mice. The results in rats confirmed an earlier study that they
had presented in 1985 showing that fluoride in the feed resulted
in precancerous growths in the mouths of rats. They also tabulated bone cancers (one sarcoma and one osteosarcoma) and
tumors (one chordoma and two chondromas) in rats fed fluoride,
but not in untreated rats. It was incredible to note that nowhere
in the text of their paper did they even refer to this data, saying
only that: *"Specific attention to target tissues revealed absence of
tumorigenic influence of fluoride."* In contradiction to their own
results, they concluded that fluoride does not cause
precancerous or cancerous changes.

While the P&G paper mentioned above did get published,
another paper reporting *"an increase in rare bone cancers among
male rats fed fluoride"*, submitted to the same journal (the
Journal of the National Cancer Institute) by the very
scientists from Battelle and the National Institute of Environmental Health Sciences that carried out the fluoride-cancer
research mandated by Congress, was rejected (September 14,
1992 issue of ***Newsweek***, p. 63).

Strategy B

Embarrassingly poor papers were published claiming that
fluoridation did not cause bone cancer. In a 1990 study by
Hrudey and coworkers, the investigators admitted: *"these data
do not allow any definitive conclusions about the role of fluoridation as a risk factor for osteosarcoma in humans. . . . with so
rare a tumor in populations the size of Calgary and Edmonton,
stable rates and statistical significance are never likely to be
achieved."*

A 1991 study by Dr. Sheila McGuire and co-workers, published in full color in the ***Journal of the American Dental
Association***, was so bad that it could be used as a classroom
example of how bad 'research' papers can get. Commenting on
this paper, Dr. Randal Harris, chairman of the Department of
Preventive Medicine of the Ohio State University, stated: *"I
briefly reviewed the article on 'Is There a Link Between Fluoridated Water and Osteosarcoma'. This is a very small study which
does not have the statistical power to find an effect, even if one exists."*

Four other papers, upon proper analysis, showed a link between fluoridation and bone cancer. Two of them (one by Dr. Robert Hoover and co-workers and another by P. D. Cohn and coworkers are discussed in Chapter 9). The results of the other two, which are tabulated below, both show net cancer increases in the fluoridated as compared to the nonfluoridated areas (F-NF).

NET BONE CANCER INCIDENCE RATES (MALE RATES MINUS FEMALE RATES) IN FLUORIDATED (F) AND NONFLUORIDATED (NF) POPULATIONS AGED 0-29 YEARS IN NEW YORK STATE

	Net Bone Cancer Rate per 100,000 Population
F	0.67
NF	0.30
F - NF	0.37

NET BONE CANCER INCIDENCE RATES (MALE RATES MINUS FEMALE RATES) IN FLUORIDATED (F) AND NONFLUORIDATED (NF) POPULATIONS

Net Bone Cancer Rate per 100,000 Population

	U.S.	Canada	U.K.	Europe	Australia New Zealand (half fluoridated)
F	0.36	0.44	0.30	—	0.20
NF	0.05	-0.10	0.27*	0.07	—
F - NF	0.31	0.54	0.03		

*According to the Tea Council, these people were drinking an average of 26 ounces of tea per day, which would lead to a consumption of 1-2 mg of fluoride per day, close to the amount consumed in a fluoridated area (the exception that proves the rule).

The USDHHS, USPHS, NTP, USEPA, P&G, and ADA have
conspired to cover up the carcinogenicity of fluoride. An April 3,
1990 letter from USEPA bureaucrat Luanna S. Wilcher to
Congressman Jon Kyl claimed *"The Procter and Gamble (P&G)
Company is also conducting a fluoride bioassay in rats and mice.
While P&G has not as yet completed their analysis, they have
informed EPA and DHHS that their preliminary results indicated no evidence of fluoride related benign or malignant bone
tumors in rats."* The NTP study, released on March 30,1990,
also cited this same report. Why would all these organizations
cite a report that none of them had seen, dealing with preliminary results of a study that had not been completed, while
disputing the results from Battelle showing a clear link between
fluoridation and cancer, the results of which they had in their
hands?

Strategy C: The Young Report

Dr. James Mason, deputy secretary of health, USDHHS, Washington, DC in 1990, assigned Frank Young to do a further
whitewash report on the NTP study.

[This is the same Mason who in 1984, as Director of the U.S.
Center for Disease Control and Assistant Surgeon General,
wrote a letter to U.S. Rep. Marvin Leath, in which he stated
that Dr. Burk (co-author of the Burk-Yiamouyiannis studies on
fluoridation and cancer) never worked for the U.S. National
Cancer Institute. According to Mason's letter, *"Dr. Dean Burk
worked for the National Cancer Institute of Canada, not the
United States."*

Demanding an apology from Dr. Mason, Dr. Burk pointed
out, *"I have never worked for the National Cancer Institute of
Canada, but I worked in the U.S. National Cancer Institute for
35 years, from May 1939 to March 1974, . . . as may readily be
confirmed by consulting* **Who's Who in America** *since 1952,*
Who's Who in the World *since its initial volume in 1971-1972,*
American Men of Science *from still earlier periods, many
similar national and international reference books, and innu-
merable articles published by me in the* **Journal of the U.S.
National Cancer Institute.** *Of the thousands of N.C.I. employ-*

ees since 1939, very few have been a scientific staff member for so long as I have. Under the circumstances, I would appreciate receiving from you a prompt statement of unreserved apology and retraction."

On November 15, 1984, and only after much pressure, Dr. Mason finally responded with a personal apology to Dr. Burk. Then on January 8, 1985, he showed his true colors again and wrote a derogatory letter about Dr. Yiamouyiannis to the Ohio Department of Health because of his opposition to fluoridation.]

In February 1991, the USDHHS came out with the Young Commission report, and on February 20, 1991, Dr. Frank Young, former FDA commissioner and then assistant undersecretary of health requested a meeting with Dr. Yiamouyiannis to discuss his study. A date of February 28, 1991 was agreed upon and on February 22, 1991, Dr. Yiamouyiannis FAXed a list of questions to be answered before the meeting. Upon receiving the FAXed questions, Dr. Young requested that the meeting be postponed to March 8, 1991 so that they would have time to prepare answers to the the questions. On March 5, 1991, Dr. Young's office contacted Dr. Yiamouyiannis to postpone the meeting again, an arrangement Dr. Yiamouyiannis felt was unacceptable since Dr. Young had more than enough time to prepare answers to the questions submitted.

On March 14, 1991, they met and Dr. Yiamouyiannis asked for point-by-point answers to the questions he had submitted. What follows are excerpts from their taped conversation:

> John Yiamouyiannis — *"Can I expect from you at some time or some date answers to some or all of the questions?"*
> Frank Young — *"I will send you some general comments on the questions that you raised. I'm not going to do a point-by-point."*
> John Yiamouyiannis — *"I don't really think that's what I'm asking for, I'm asking really for specific answers to specific questions and if you have any problems with any questions, that's fine with me. If you say we could not answer this question because we could not understand it."*

> Frank Young — *"To the ones I feel that we would be able to answer, I'll try to provide some general answers to. What I will not do is go point-by-point-by-point because I don't want you and I to be pen pals forever."*
> John Yiamouyiannis — *"No. As a matter fact, I was hoping to have the answers to the questions before I came up here, as we talked about in our telephone conversation on the 22nd [of February, 1991]. . . . I feel that a person, or anyone who signs off on a report like this is responsible for the accuracy of these statements".*
> Frank Young — *"There is no question about that. The thing you have to realize is that I have zero staff."*

Dr. Yiamouyiannis also asked him about a number of crucial concerns that should have been addressed in the report:

> John Yiamouyiannis — *"The osteomas showed a dose-dependent relationship with fluoride."*
> Frank Young — Referring to osteomas said *"I'm not sure they are tumors."*
> [Webster's 3rd defines osteoma as *"a benign tumor composed of bone tissue"*]
> John Yiamouyiannis — *"I did go through the Hoover study and so far as I can read . . . in fluoridated areas, the osteosarcoma [bone cancer] rate was about 30-40% higher . . . "*
> Frank Young — *"That is correct"*

Dr. Young was asked how he felt with regard to his justification for disregarding the higher osteosarcoma rate found by the NCI study:

> John Yiamouyiannis — *"How do you feel, Frank?"*
> Frank Young — *"I felt with absolute certainty in my belly, after getting the questions answered, that I could accept this."*
> John Yiamouyiannis — *"The concern I also brought to you was that you accepted the NTP study [on cancer]."*
> Frank Young — *"Yes. And that's a valid concern. I'm going to get that report and read it. . . We relied upon the NTP peer review. . . We did not, as a committee, go back, to my knowledge, and pull the raw data."*

Dr. Yiamouyiannis asked him about a number of errors in the report.

> John Yiamouyiannis — *"Let's talk about one enzyme in particular, acetylcholinesterase."*
> Frank Young — *"Yeah."*
> John Yiamouyiannis — *"Which you said fluoride affects this and other enzymes by binding to the metal cofactor. Now acetylcholinesterase . . . does not have any metal cofactor."*
> Frank Young — *"I will look at that particular work . . ."*

There were only two specific original studies cited in the report purporting to compare fluoridated and nonfluoridated areas that were presented to support the claim that fluoridation reduces tooth decay. One of them was a 1955 study comparing two areas that were fluoridated, Grand Rapids and Muskegon, Michigan (the other study cited had too few students to provide any meaningful conclusions).

> John Yiamouyiannis — *"You already admitted that . . . Muskegon . . . was fluoridated as a matter of fact in 1951 and so you agree that that was at least some type of mistake — it was a mistake there in calling that nonfluoridated."*
> Frank Young — *"I would agree that it was originally cited as a control [nonfluoridated] community and was fluoridated . . ."*

Regarding implications within the report that items such as fluoridated toothpaste, not fluoridated water, is responsible for the high rates of dental fluorosis in the United States, Dr. Yiamouyiannis made a suggestion.

> John Yiamouyiannis — *"If you really believe that people get so much fluoride from toothpaste . . ."*
> Frank Young — *"Yeah . . ."*
> John Yiamouyiannis — *". . . then you and I ought to go out to the public, hold a joint press conference, and say we can stop fluoridating, you can swallow your toothpaste and get all the fluoride you want."*

> Frank Young — *"I'll tell you why we won't, because the poor people brush with bicarbonate of soda. . . ."*
> John Yiamouyiannis — *"Do you have studies on that too?"*
> Frank Young — *"No. no. no."*

And Dr. Yiamouyiannis asked him about the bias and cover up in the report bringing special attention to the fact that a substantial portion of his committee members were fluoridation supporters.

> John Yiamouyiannis — *"There's Stephen Corbin . . . a major promoter of fluoridation."*
> Frank Young — *"Stephen is a biased person. . . I would consider he was a profluoridationist."*
> John Yiamouyiannis —*"We have Lawrence Furman."*
> Frank Young — *"I did not know where he was at the beginning but I would consider he is a person that has promoted fluorides."*
> John Yiamouyiannis —*"Not only that but he is head of the division of the Centers of Disease Control which actually politically supports fluoridation nationally."*
> Frank Young — *"Yes, that's correct."*
> John Yiamouyiannis — *"Hoel."*
> Frank Young — *"Hoel has no position on fluoride."*
> John Yiamouyiannis — *"He's taken a very seriously pro position on fluoride and I have a letter from him."*
> Frank Young — *"OK, I am sorry. That I did not know."*
> John Yiamouyiannis — *"Vernon Houk, who is Furman's predecessor. Harald Loe, who is the former director of the NIDR."*
> Frank Young — *"Oh, yes."*
> John Yiamouyiannis — *"Here we have a group of people . . . who are highly profluoridation . . . "*
> Frank Young — *"But there are some that were not though in fairness."*
> John Yiamouyiannis — *"Oh, but there were none that were against it. No one against it."*
> Frank Young — *"I would say of the people that were*

there, there were not any that were against it. I would agree with that."
John Yiamouyiannis — *"But there were some that were for it."*
Frank Young — *"There were some that were for it."*
John Yiamouyiannis — *"All I'm saying is that you wouldn't choose a jury this way if your life was at stake."*
John Yiamouyiannis — *"But you see these are the things that concern me if these people were experts who were on your committee ... that this whole list of people that were supposed to be experts ... allowed somewhere around 50-60 serious errors to go through."*
Frank Young — *"John, I would only say this in defense of errors going through on any thing. ... I would not ever say that there is not a mistake in there."*
John Yiamouyiannis — *"Errors can be random or they can be directed. When errors are directed, I have a real problem."*
Frank Young — *"... I don't believe it's a directed ... "*
John Yiamouyiannis — *"These errors are made continually in the report in the direction of trying to indicate that fluoride isn't harmful when it is."*
Frank Young — *"John, if it's made in a direction that indicates that fluoridation isn't harmful, it wasn't deliberate to the best of my knowledge."*
Kay Turner — *"Without the balance, which I believe John said was lacking, it's going to be easy to have your neutral parties fall into the pro camp."*
Frank Young — *"That is the bias that I was afraid of."*
John Yiamouyiannis — *"Now the Public Health Service has been on record since 1950 ... "*
Frank Young — *"I know."*
John Yiamouyiannis — *"... as what?"*
Frank Young — *"I knew you would ask."*
John Yiamouyiannis — *"... as what?"*
Frank Young — *"... as supporting fluoridation."*
John Yiamouyiannis — *"OK. Now they come out with a report supporting fluoridation, is there any surprise? What's the surprise?"*

In the Young Report, the section on fluoride and tooth decay leaves out data from the largest and the most recent studies on fluoride and tooth decay, including those of Colquhoun (1990) on approximately 60,000 schoolchildren, Yiamouyiannis (1990) on approximately 39,000 schoolchildren, and Hildebolt, et al. (1989) on approximately 6000 schoolchildren.

Studies are cited for confirmation of the 'benefits' of fluoride which actually contradict any alleged benefit of fluoride. For example, the report cites a study by Disney and co-workers as supporting the school-based fluoride mouthrinse program instigated by the National Institute of Dental Research (NIDR). In fact, the study by Disney presents data showing that the fluoride mouthrinse program does not work. They even addressed the disparity between their findings and those of the NIDR studies by stating *"Since the FMR [fluoride mouthrinse program] results were in direct contrast to those of previous NIDR supported studies and existing public health practices, it was quite natural that the earliest reaction came from the NIDR"*.

In the section on fluoride and cancer, the lead paragraph claims that animal studies done before 1970 relevant to fluoridation and cancer were negative. This is untrue, as can be seen by the studies of Taylor (1954), Herskowitz and Norton (1963), and Taylor and Taylor (1965).

The report ignored the data from Battelle Laboratories that was returned to the NTP and covered over the most significant results of the NTP study.

The section of the report on cancer epidemiology, similar to the report's section on fluoride and tooth decay, is inaccurate. Claims were made that the studies showing a link between fluoridation and cancer did not correct for age, race, and sex, when in fact they did.

The report refused to point out the admitted errors of studies by Hoover, et al., Doll and Kinlen, and Oldham and Newell, which, when corrected, led to the finding of a link between fluoridation and cancer.

The report ignored Dr. Yiamouyiannis's most recent epidemiological studies showing a link between fluoridation and cancer.

The report cites reviews concluding that fluoride is not linked to cancer, but ignores findings confirming a link, including the report of the Environment Ministry of Quebec and the report of the chief toxicologist of the state of Virginia.

The report hides in its appendix (on Table C-2) the incriminating data of Leverett and Segretto showing dental fluorosis rates of 25-40% in fluoridated areas as compared to levels of under 10% in nonfluoridated areas, while highlighting only those findings showing a minimal relationship between fluoridation and dental fluorosis in the main text.

The report claims that *"recent studies of conventional design to evaluate developmental toxicity of sodium fluoride have not been reported"*, when in fact Iarez, et al. (1981) showed that fluoride was teratogenic in rats and Zhang and Zhang (1983) showed that fluoride caused birth defects in fish.

The report makes unsubstantiated statements regarding water fluoridation and kidney problems, gastrointestinal problems, hypersensitivity, immunologic effects, and crippling skeletal fluorosis.

Another Bogus Report

As mentioned in the previous chapter, the EPA had contracted with ICAIR Life Systems to put out a fluoride cover-up report in 1985. In 1991, they again used ICAIR Life Systems — this time to do a literature search on fluoride. Dr. John Beaver, a researcher for ICAIR Life Systems who worked on the 1991 project, admitted that he was instructed to select only certain reports and exclude others. These reports were sent to the EPA who forwarded them on to the Subcommittee on Risk Assessment of Ingested Fluoride of the National Academy of Sciences for another 'independent' report.

Of the eight members on this subcommittee, three are among the most notorious fluoridation promoters. These include Dr. James W. Bawden, of the University of North Carolina, who has threatened Dr. Yiamouyiannis with physical violence, Dr. Brian Burt, of the University of Michigan, who has tried to stop Dr. Yiamouyiannis from presenting papers before scientific groups, and Dr. Kenneth Cantor, who coauthored (with Robert Hoover) the article trying to cover up the link between fluoride and bone cancer; Cantor's study was published in the Young Report. Two are well-known fluoridation promoters: Dr. Steven Levy of the University of Iowa and Gary Whitford of the Medical College of Georgia.[26] The National Academy of Sciences subcommittee's principal scientist is Dr. Marvin Schneiderman, who was a primary figure in the original attempts by the National Cancer Institute to cover up the fluoride-cancer link. With a biased list of references, with five of eight members of the subcommittee already 'in the bag', and with a staff scientist who has been accused of perjury in his attempts to defend fluoridation (see Chapter 20), what do you expect?

---

[26] the remaining members include Bernard M. Wagner of Wagner Associates, Dr. Daniel Krewski, an administrator with Health and Welfare of Canada, and Ernest Eugene McConnell of Raleigh, NC.

Chapter 19

The Extended Conspiracy: Their Evil Network

If it is evil for the United States Public Health Service to conduct experiments on 400 black men at Tuskegee Institute and 'study' their suffering while watching over 100 of them die in misery of syphilis, without helping with the drugs that could have cured their illnesses, if it is evil for the Atomic Energy Commission, alias the Department of Energy, to purposely release gigantic amounts of radioactivity into the atmosphere around the Hanford nuclear facility in Washington State to see what it might do to the health of people living in the area, if it is evil for the American Dental Association and the United States Public Health Service to work together to continue to dictate the use of silver/mercury amalgam fillings despite the harmful effects they are having on millions of people, if it is evil for Beech-Nut to malnourish millions of babies by selling colored sugar water as apple juice, etc., etc., . . . then we've got a network of evil in this country that we can't hide from any longer.

Normally one would expect the state and national environmental protection agencies to step in and stop fluoride pollution of our air and water. Certainly one would expect the Food and Drug Administration[27] to set regulations limiting the amount of fluoride contamination of phosphates used for animal feeds and fertilizers. Certainly one would expect the state and national public health services to stop the purposeful addition of fluoride to our drinking water.

But they don't. Their behavior on other issues of vital importance is briefly mentioned here to indicate that their treatment of the fluoride problem is not an isolated incident.

---

[27] Dr. Frank Fazzari of the FDA has indicated that because he has found that FDA has no studies showing that fluoride tablets and drops are either safe or effective, the FDA would be taking them off the market shortly.

CDC and the Swine Flu Vaccine Fiasco

Many are aware of the swine flu fiasco that was promoted by the Centers for Disease Control (CDC) and other branches of the U.S. Public Health Service. Due to this government-sponsored health fraud, 40,000,000 Americans were vaccinated against a disease which never existed — with a vaccine that would not have worked even if the disease existed. Dr. Anthony Morris, a U.S. Food and Drug Administration scientist who sounded a warning of the hazards and uselessness of the swine flu program before it was instituted, was fired as a result of his warning.

Even before the vaccine was administered, the public health service realized that the vaccine would produce fevers in about 10% of those injected. This comes to a figure of 4,000,000 people who suffered the needless pain and discomfort of a fever. A conservative estimate of 10,000 deaths may be attributed to this program. The swine flu vaccine has also been linked to approximately 1000 known victims of the Guillan-Barre syndrome, a disease in which the body's own immune system is stimulated to attack nerves, resulting in paralysis.

And what about Dr. David Sencer who was responsible for the promotion of this disastrous program at CDC? He went on to promote fluoridation as the health commissioner of New York City.

IARC and OSHA:
Their Involvement in the Formaldehyde Cover-Up

Agency scientists may express their scientific opinion *"provided they're not in conflict with agency policy. Everybody follows a policy."* With this excuse, top bureaucrats at the Occupational Safety and Health Administration (OSHA) tried to dismiss Dr. Peter Infante, director of OSHA's office of carcinogen identification and classification, for pointing out that formaldehyde causes cancer.

According to the July 27, 1981 issue of **Chemical & Engineering News**, Dr. Infante wrote a letter to Dr. John Higginson, director of the International Agency for Research on

Cancer (IARC), disagreeing with the decision of an IARC committee to water down the cancer-causing potential of formaldehyde.

"*According to IARC criteria*", Infante wrote, "*there appears to have been sufficient experimental evidence to regard formaldehyde as carcinogenic in animals.*" In this letter, Dr. Infante cited a Current Intelligence Bulletin (CIB) on formaldehyde as an "*important document assessing formaldehyde's cancer-causing potential.*"

As a result, Higginson wrote to OSHA director Thorne G. Auchter complaining that: "*Dr. Infante's letter casts aspersions on the competence and objectivity of the working group of IARC.*" Subsequently, the Formaldehyde Institute, an umbrella organization for makers and users of formaldehyde, contacted high level bureaucrats at OSHA, who later recommended that OSHA not release the CIB report on formaldehyde and who initiated formal proceedings to dismiss Infante.

During sworn testimony before a Congressional subcommittee investigating this affair, OSHA director Thorne Auchter and Dr. Bailus Walker argued as to which one was responsible for seeking Dr. Infante's dismissal. Neither was willing to take the blame. Mr. Auchter did admit, however, to scuttling the CIB report, saying, "*I lack confidence in the data for regulatory purposes.*" But he also added that he had not studied that data. "*It would be a waste of time*", he said. "*I wouldn't understand it.*"

IARC and NCI:
Their Involvement in the Benzene Cover-Up

The August 8, 1982 issue of the *Houston Post* reports that IARC purposely deleted a crucial sentence in its report on benzene. According to the *Post*:

"*The sentence, of concern to 500,000 U.S. workers exposed to benzene, had stated that lifetime benzene workers, under currently permitted conditions, might suffer triple the normal rate of leukemia.*"

The killer of the sentence, Dr. Lorenzo Tomatis of the International Agency for Research on Cancer in Lyon, France, has

confessed. But he appears to have had two American accom-
plices, one a usual suspect and the other a real shocker. The
usual suspect is the Washington-based Chemical Manufacturers
Association [CMA], representing U.S. chemical companies. The
other shocker is the National Cancer Institute's [NCI] Division
of Cancer Cause and Prevention, which, according to documents
released by Rep. David Obey, D. Wis., joined with them to get
the benzene-leukemia finding killed.

"The CMA found an ally in Dr. Richard H. Adamson, director of the Cancer Cause and Prevention Unit of the National
Cancer Institute based in Bethesda, MD. The institute provides
$3 million of the multinational IARC's overall $13 million
budget. Moreover, according to IARC officials, Adamson's office
controls half the $694,500 budget item that enables Tomatis to
invite the world's leading researchers to travel, meet and dine in
Lyon and publish papers on major cancer issues. . . a subordi-
nate of Adamson's, Dr. Herman Kraybill, who oversees Tomatis'
contract with NCI, successfully urged a dinner in Lyon at which
he and Tomatis discussed benzene with Dr. Jesse Norris of the
CMA."

This is the same Dr. Adamson that was on the Frank Young
Committee that issued the whitewash report on fluoride in
1991. And this is the same Herman Kraybill who was placed in
charge of the NTP study to see if fluoride caused cancer and
referred to it as "the final study to confirm negativity of fluoride
ion in carcinogenesis." In view of Dr. Kraybill's liaison position
between the NCI and IARC, it came as no surprise that, in 1982,
IARC came out with a whitewash report claiming no link between fluoridation and cancer.

The Evil Conspiracy

The National Institute of Dental Research (NIDR), working in
cooperation with the United States Environmental Protection
Agency, the Centers of Disease Control, the Food and Drug
Administration, and other divisions of the Department of Health
and Human Services, the Department of Defense, the American
Dental Association, Procter and Gamble, various universities,
most notably the University of Minnesota and the University of

Rochester, the National Academy of Sciences, and others have served as the front group for the real villains, the fluoride-polluting industries, the junk food industries, and the pharmaceutical-cosmetic industry.

The fluoride-polluting industries (steel, coal burning, phosphate and phosphate fertilizer, aluminum, ceramics, hydrofluoric acid production, petrochemical, glass manufacture, frit manufacture, cement manufacture, nonferrous metals, uranium, and others) benefit from fluoridation in two ways.

First, as Rebecca Hammer, U.S. Environmental Protection Agency deputy assistant administrator pointed out in 1983, fluoride-polluting industries can get paid for using public drinking waters as a sewer for their toxic waste products.

"In regard to the use of fluosilicic acid as a source of fluoride for fluoridation, this agency regards such use as an ideal environmental solution to a long-standing problem. By recovering by-product fluosilicic acid from fertilizer manufacturing, water and air pollution are minimized, and water utilities have a low-cost source of fluoride available to them."

Most importantly, now that fluoride is purposely added to public drinking waters with claims that it is beneficial to health and safe, it is more difficult for people to complain about it when polluting industries belch it out into the air and dump it into our waterways. The indiscriminate and careless handling of fluoride allows companies such as Exxon, U.S. Steel, and ALCOA to make tens of billions of dollars of extra profit at the expense of hundreds of millions of Americans.

After all, if fluoride is safe and good, how can industries be successfully sued in court for damage to human health from their pollution? And how can strict government regulation of fluoride pollution — very expensive to industry — be enforced?

The junk food industries, who sell their sugar-laden, tooth-decay-producing 'treats' to children during the cavity-prone years, can continue to fraudulently assert that it's all right because fluoride in the water will prevent the tooth decay that their wares would otherwise cause.

And the pharmaceutical and cosmetic industries can continue to reap windfall profits selling fluoride tablets and drops which are unsafe and ineffective in treating tooth decay or osteoporosis, as well as rinses, gels, and toothpastes, which have a minimal effect on tooth decay but, in many cases, contain a lethal dose of fluoride.

Even the American Medical Association, conned into promoting fluoridation by the American Dental Association, continues to play along with this charade to save their reputation, rather than to admit they were wrong and let the public know that physicians can make mistakes.

Over the years, the conspiracy has entwined others 'a la Bernays' (see Chapter 16). Note how the lies and deception are passed on like a plague.

Consumer Reports

With the help of fluoride promoters, **Consumer Reports** prepared and published a two-part article on fluoride in its July and August 1978 issues. The writer of these articles was Mr. Joseph Botta. Mr. Botta holds a Master of Arts Degree in English, but no scientific degree. In this article he passed along the same lies and slander used by the promoters to the trusting readers of **Consumer Reports**.

The **Consumer Reports** article on fluoridation is the most artfully written piece incorporating the lies and slander necessary to discredit the research and personalities of scientists showing that fluoridation is harmful. It is by far the Number One article distributed by the government bureaucrats in their promotion of fluoridation. This is not because government bureaucrats are not skillful liars. It is because, by having their spoon-fed material rewritten and published by a 'consumer' magazine, their lies become more believable. Dr. William Bock of the Centers for Disease Control thought it was so good that he ordered 10,000 reprints and paid for them with federal tax dollars. The American Dental Association gave Mr. Botta an award for writing it.

This **Consumer Reports** article was used by U.S. Public Health Service bureaucrats to provide a 'scientific' foundation for their views on fluoridation. The situation has become ludicrous. For example, Dr. Vernon Houk, the director of the Environmental Center for Health of the Centers for Disease Control, traveled all the way from Atlanta, Georgia, to St. Paul, Minnesota, to give his 'expert' testimony by reading from the ***Consumer Reports*** article.

The 'Big Lie' in this article and the phrase most often quoted from it is the claim that *"The simple truth is that there's no 'scientific controversy' over the safety of fluoridation."* In 1990, Dr. Edward Groth III, the technical director for ***Consumer Reports***, nullified this claim by stating: *"The point is that this is a legitimate scientific controversy. Proponents of fluoridation insist that there are no grounds for controversy at all, and with that, I totally disagree."* This hasn't stopped proponents from quoting the same phrase to this day.

Who is Stephen Barrett?

Dr. Stephen Barrett, a psychiatrist, helped in the preparation of the 1978 ***Consumer Reports*** article and of the 1988 book ***Abuse of the Scientific Literature in an Antifluoridation Pamphlet*** (see Chapter 17). He has close ties with the American Dental Association, the American Medical Association, and the U.S. Public Health Service. He is a recipient of the FDA award for 'quack-busting' and is a coauthor, along with William Jarvis and others, of the 1993 book ***Readers' Guide to Alternative Health Methods***, published by the American Medical Association. In this book, he cites, and gives summaries of, the two publications mentioned above to inform his readers about fluoridation. He is a science and editorial adviser to the American Council of Science and Health.

A glimpse into his character can be gained through his habitual use of words to mean their exact opposite. For example, in an article entitled 'Poison Mongers', Dr. Barrett refers to people who are trying to stop the addition of fluoride, a poison, to the water supply as poison-mongers. Now a monger is one who sells something, e.g. a fishmonger is a person who sells fish. Therefore, it is quite evident that a poison-monger is a person who sells poison. Thus, one opposed to having fluoride added to the water supply is exactly the opposite of a poison-monger. The word usage of Dr. Barrett is comparable to the process called 'Newspeak' described in George Orwell's ***1984***, where what is true becomes false and what is false becomes true. The first few paragraphs of Dr. Barrett's article 'Poison-Mongers' is the best example of how Dr. Barrett has used 'Newspeak'.

> *"In hundreds of American communities citizens have voted against healthier teeth.*
> *"Why?*
> *"They were confused — by poison-mongers.*
> *"These alarmists in our society are using confusion and a scare vocabulary as weapons against fluoridation. They are cheating all of us, but especially our children.*
> *"The benefits of fluoridation are supported by 10,000 scientific studies which prove the poison-mongers are wrong.*
> *"What do the poison-mongers say?*
> *"Instead of telling you that fluoride is found naturally in all water, they call it a 'pollutant'.*
> *"Instead of telling you that fluoride is a nutrient essential to life, they call it a 'poison'.*
> *"Instead of the big truth, that fluoridation has never harmed anyone, they tell the big lie and say it causes hundreds of ailments."*

This article was published in newspapers across the country and was printed in the November 1976 issue of the ***Journal of the American Dental Association***. It has also been used by the U.S. Public Health Service in its 'education' of Congressmen and in its campaign to get various areas around the country fluoridated.

A closer look into Dr. Barrett's personality can be obtained by examining his correspondence in 1972 with a group of people in Minnesota interested in stopping fluoridation. On March 8, 1972, Dr. Barrett wrote to one of these people, saying:

> *"I read your letter in **Prevention** [magazine] with some interest. There have been other attempts to defeat the fluoridationists in court — but most have failed. Before investing money, I would like to have full details of what you plan.*
> *"Thanks, Stephen J. Barrett, M.D."*

In another letter to these people, dated April 4, 1972, Dr. Barrett wrote:

> *"Thank you for your recent telephone call. I am sorry that I could not immediately make the financial commitment which you requested. I know how enthusiastic you are and did not want to raise your hopes until I had a chance to discuss the matter with my group.*
>
> *"I am part of a group which is vitally concerned about fluoridation and which has raised a considerable amount of money. We are not yet sure whether it would be more practical to lobby or to go to court in Pennsylvania. The reason your lawsuit interests us is because it might be more practical for us to join your effort rather than go it alone.*
>
> *"Thus we would need to have a detailed, written description of the plans of your suit. Our attorneys would then be in a position to study how it would effect Pa. law and also to estimate the chances of your suit being successful. We would also need some detail as to how the Attorney General's favorable attitude will be used to advantage without this becoming apparent to the American Dental Association.*
>
> *"We realize you are hesitant to say too much about your plans. On the other hand, we could not make a total commitment unless we had full knowledge of what we would be getting for our investment. We realize this asks alot of you. On the other hand, we think we have a lot to offer.*
>
> *"You may be assured that whatever information you send us will be handled with appropriate discretion.*
>
> *"Sincerely yours, Stephen Barrett, M.D."*

On April 12, 1972, he wrote another letter to Miss Mary Bernhardt, the person at the American Dental Association responsible for promoting fluoridation, and related the following:

"Dear Miss Bernhardt:

"At about 6:20 this evening, I received another phone call from Mike Liptak, the organizer of MOFF [Minnesotans Opposed to Forced Fluoridation]. He said that at 4:30, Judge Gordon McRae ordered an injunction 'to keep the fluoride out of Brainerd.'

"He said that there were 1500 people who watched the trial and that the judge had cautioned them about becoming emotional. They were very quiet. The case presented by MOFF included an affidavit from Dr. Waldbott. The attorney-general of Minnesota defended and was given 'five days for rebuttal.' According to Mr. Liptak, who again said he went to school with the attorney general, the attorney general said he 'would not furnish a rebuttal'. He merely stated that the new Minnesota law required fluoridation.

"Mr. Liptak added that there was an additional legal action scheduled for September. In about two weeks, 500 local citizens were planning to gather at a meeting where the vice-president of a local bank would get from them '3 year notes for $50 each' to help finance the suit. He expected that such mass action would not get them much publicity in **Prevention** *magazine and the National Health Federation. It was their plan to seek further injunctions of this type with eventual overturning of the new state laws. He again asked me for a contribution, even a token one. He added that there might be money left over for use in another state such as Pennsylvania.*

"On 5/14, Dr. Gross will try to contact leaders of the profluoridation forces in the Minnesota Dental Society and will also call the American Dental Association attorney. We have Mr. Liptak's confidence and hope to continue to use it to our advantage. Perhaps the dental society should consider entering the suit as a guardian of the children. It might also be helpful if some quick way could be devised to dissuade the Brainerd residents from their imminent investment in foolishness.

"Best wishes, Stephen Barrett, M.D."

Ironically, Dr. Barrett is a co-founder of the National Council Against Health Fraud.

Subsequently, he and Mary Bernhardt got together and published a book called *The Health Robbers*, in which they refer to those opposing fluoridation as health robbers. Excerpts from this book, which consist primarily of the substance of his poison-monger article, were reprinted in newspapers around the country, as well as in *Family Health Magazine*.

Teaming up with others of his kind, including Drs. Thomas Jukes, Warren Winklestein, and Joel M. Boriskin, Dr. Barrett complained about and tried to prevent Dr. Yiamouyiannis from speaking before the Faculty Club of the University of California, Berkeley. Together they claimed that Dr. Yiamouyiannis was some disreputable person not deserving a forum at the University of California campus.

In another action, Dr. Barrett, Dr. Boriskin and Dr. William Jarvis, who also is on the board of the National Council Against Health Fraud, wrote letters of complaint to the National News Council concerning an article published in the *National Enquirer* which pointed out that higher cancer risks were associated with fluoridation.

An indication of how Barrett's 'Newspeak' is passed down the line to local dentists is evident from the experience Dr. Yiamouyiannis had when he was called in by local residents of St. Charles, Missouri for a debate on fluoridation. When Dr. Michael Garvey, a local dentist, heard that Dr. Yiamouyiannis was going to be the opposition speaker, he refused to participate in the debate.

According to the November 12, 1982 *St. Charles Post*: *"Dr. Garvey said American Dental Association Officials had told him, 'running up against Dr. Yiamouyiannis is not recommended'. The man is well-known as an antifluoridation speaker, Dr. Garvey said. 'This guy is a terror.'"*

The Saint Charles Council proceeded to hold the debate in the absence of Dr. Garvey. In an attempt to impugn the integrity of Dr. Yiamouyiannis, Dr. Garvey released a statement to the press claiming that:

> *"Yiamouyiannis is viewed in the bona fide scientific
> medical and dental community as a walking example of
> scientific fraud. The problem is, that he's so smooth in his
> presentation that the average person without a scientific
> background will be snowed and is likely to believe his
> every word.*
>
> *"This Yiamouyiannis is a 'poisonmonger,' according
> to experts in the bona fide scientific community. Instead
> of telling you that fluoride is found naturally in all water,
> he will tell you that it's a 'pollutant'. Instead of telling you
> that fluoride is a nutrient essential to life, he will call it a
> 'poison'. Instead of the big truth, that water fluoridation
> has never harmed anyone, he will espouse untruths and
> say it causes cancer and hundreds of ailments."*

If this sounds familiar, it is probably because the words are
merely parroting Dr. Barrett's 'Newspeak'.

Academic Freedom?

In a related action, Dr. Jukes and his 'gang' went after Dr. John
Neilands, professor of biochemistry at the University of California, Berkeley, for taking a public stand against fluoridation.
They complained to his department head and sought to have
him expelled from his professional society. Dr. James Petrakis,
the investigator sent by the society, concluded that Dr. Neilands
*"is a reputable scientist . . is politically active and loves to chal-
lenge the status quo. In my view, he is usually right. He is no
kook."*

Wendy Lewis, a graduate student in nutrition at the University of California, Berkeley, invited Dr. John Lee, a local physician and fluoridation opponent, on campus to present his views
on fluoridation. As a result, Dr. Jukes wrote to Ms. Lewis: *"you
are not airing a controversy, you are merely giving an opportunity for misinformation to be presented."* In a letter to her
department head, he wrote: *"What has gone awry in the guid-
ance of your students? Why does the department not cancel the
invitation of Dr. Lee?"*

Commenting on the situation, Dr. Petrakis said: *"I do not
know Thomas Jukes, nor do I want to. In my opinion, his raging*

*intolerance of contrary views — even those that might be errone-
ous — is most unbecoming to an academic man. His Scriptural
attitude on the issue of fluoridation, to use his own language,
'brings disgrace on the name of biochemistry,' which is supposed
to be an investigative science, not a set of immutable beliefs
chiseled in stone."*

Government Funds for Intimidation and Propaganda

An example of the use of government funds for intimidation was
reported in the September 1, 1978 issue of the ***Kansas City
Times***. The ***Times*** carried statements made by Cora Leukhart,
a former low-level bureaucrat (under the supervision of Dr.
William Bock) at the Centers for Disease Control. While attending a conference sponsored by the Environmental Protection
Agency, she stated that: *"If we adopt a national health plan,
those communities which will not fluoridate shouldn't be subsi-
dized."* According to the paper, *"she referred several times to a
two-part article in the July and August [1978] editions of **Consumer Reports**."*

An example of the use of government funds for propaganda
was reported in the September 19, 1980 issue of ***The (Portland) Oregonian***. The ***Oregonian*** reported:

*"An investigator for the Criminal Division of the Oregon
attorney general's office has recommended criminal prosecution
of two Multnomah County administrators for allegedly violating
a state law forbidding electioneering on public time, **The Oregonian** has learned. Subjects of the investigation are David
Lawrence, director of the county's Department of Human Services, and Robert Isman, director of dental services."*

In addition, these county administrators were issued a $55,000
'fluoride education grant' to promote fluoridation by the section
of the Centers for Disease Control headed by Dr. Bock. This
grant was used for full-page ads to influence an election on
whether Portland, the largest city in Multnomah County, would
fluoridate. Similar attempts to illegally influence the outcome of
fluoridation elections with federal tax dollars have been made by
other government agencies.

The Government — A Conduit for Evil

In October of 1985, Dr. Yiamouyiannis was called in to help three local groups of citizens in San Antonio to help stop fluoridation. The City Council had voted earlier that year to add fluoride to the water and the three citizens' groups had since gotten enough signatures to put the issue on the November ballot.

Mayor Henry Cisneros, a leading contender for the vice presidential spot with Walter Mondale in 1984 and a presidential hopeful himself, was putting his reputation on the line in support of fluoridation. Having won the last mayoral election with over 90% of the vote and having the endorsements and financial support of many of the influential segments of the community, it seemed as if Mayor Cisneros would have no difficulty getting fluoridation into San Antonio. In short, because of a line-up of some very sharp citizens opposed to fluoridation and because of a spontaneous yet well-organized effort on their part, San Antonians defeated fluoridation on November 5, 1985 by a vote of 52% to 48%.

During the campaign, efforts were made to keep Dr. Yiamouyiannis, one of their chosen spokespersons, off of a television debate scheduled for prime time against Mayor Cisneros and a local physician. The excuse — Dr. Yiamouyiannis was not a local resident and only local residents would be allowed to debate.

As a result, Dr. Yiamouyiannis, who was running for political office in Ohio, withdrew from the election, notified the board of elections as well as the media in Ohio, registered to vote in San Antonio, and returned to the television station with voter registration card at 5 p.m. At that point, the television station agreed they could have no further objections to his appearing in the debate. By the following morning, Mayor Cisneros had withdrawn from the debate, deciding instead to send his wife into the debate to take the heat.

That afternoon, Dr. Yiamouyiannis received a call from his wife (still back in Ohio) saying that some suspiciously acting woman had stopped by, asking about him but refusing to identify herself. After taking down this person's license plate number and tracing it to a Patricia Payne from Columbus, Ohio, Mrs. Yiamouyiannis received a call one hour later from a profluoridation columnist from San Antonio who related a conversation he had had with a Patty Payne from the attorney general's office in Ohio. Apparently, a whole web of cruddy politicians from Texas to Ohio and back again were using tax-payers' monies to (1) intimidate Mrs. Yiamouyiannis and (2) try to show that Dr. Yiamouyiannis was violating some election laws.

The Death of Science?

Concerned about the impact of reports of high mortality in fluoridated areas, John Small arranged a meeting with members of the National Heart, Lung and Blood Institute (NHBLI). As a result of the meeting, Dr. A. Richey Sharrett, a public health physician, began yet another study to prove that mortality rates were not higher in fluoridated areas. Of all the studies instigated by Mr. Small, this one was worst. Dr. Sharrett and his co-workers, Drs. Eugene Rogot, Manning Feinleib and Richard Fabsitz, left out 80-90% of the relevant data.

The quality of thinking that went into this study is exemplified by Dr. Sharrett's testimony in a fluoridation court case in Scotland. It was shown that the study by Dr. Sharrett and co-workers did nothing more than measure random variation and was not relevant to the question as to whether fluoride caused cancer. In defending his study against this criticism, Dr. Sharrett claimed that the extremely low cancer death rate in Miami Beach in 1950 was not due to random variation. He claimed that the reason that the cancer death rate in Miami Beach was so extremely low was that *"people who retire to the warm climate of Florida are people who are able to do so, whose health permits them to. Anyone who is likely to be losing weight and seeing a doctor frequently. . ."* It was then pointed out that this could not be true since cancer death rates throughout Florida were uniformly much higher.

In another equally unsupportable statement, Dr. Sharrett claimed that the cancer death rate of Beverly Hills in 1950 was extremely low because *"these people have all the advantages."* In response to his claim, the Queen's Counsel cross-examined Dr. Sharrett as follows:

> Queen's Counsel: *"Well, they have all the advantages. Well now, that is so far as 1950 is concerned. Did they lose their advantages in 1960?"*
>
> Dr. Sharrett: *"I don't know what happened to Beverly Hills in 1960, I have never been there."*
>
> Queen's Counsel: *"You know what happened in 1950 because they had all the advantages, and I am asking you did they lose these advantages by 1960?"*
>
> Dr. Sharrett: *"I do know that some years back Beverly Hills was reputed to be the place of movie stars; I don't know whether it has changed in recent times or not."*
>
> Queen's Counsel: *"But you were able to say these people had all the advantages in 1950, have you any reason to believe that your information to that effect was information which did not apply also to 1960."*
>
> Dr. Sharrett: *"No, I don't have the detail to talk about what may or may not have transpired in Beverly Hills."*
>
> Queen's Counsel: *"Well, let's see what did transpire in Beverly Hills so far as 1960 was concerned. In 1950 I think they had a cancer SMR of .650?"*
>
> Dr. Sharrett: *"Are you asking me about that mortality ratio?"*
>
> Queen's Counsel: *"Yes, .650 in 1950?"*
>
> Dr. Sharrett: *"Yes."*
>
> Queen's Counsel: *"And that SMR doubled in 1960 to 1.022?"*
>
> Dr. Sharrett: *"Yes, I see that."*
>
> Queen's Counsel: *"And climbed to 1.129 in 1970?"*
>
> Dr. Sharrett: *"Yes."*
>
> Queen's Counsel: *"Now, how were you able to suggest, in light of that evidence, that the low mortality ratio in Beverly Hills is attributable to the advantages which the people, lucky enough to live in that community, obtained?"*

With regard to science at the EPA, Dr. Robert J. Carton, Vice-President of the EPA's union of professional workers and scientists, made the following observations:

> *"The fluoride in drinking water standard, or Recommended Maximum Contaminant Level (RMCL) for fluoride, published by EPA in the **Federal Register** on Nov. 14, 1985, is a classic case of political interference with science. The regulation is a fraudulent statement by the Federal Government that 4 milligram per liter (mg/l) of fluoride in drinking water is safe with an adequate margin of safety. There is evidence that critical information in the scientific and technical support documents used to develop the standard was falsified by the Department of Health and Human Services and the Environmental Protection Agency to protect a long-standing public health policy."*
>
> *"Data showing positive correlations between fluoride exposure and genetic effects in almost all of the laboratory tests were discounted. By selective use of data, they fit science to the desired outcome."*

And what about science at the National Institute of Dental Research? In 1978, Dr. George Martin, while testifying in a court case in Pennsylvania that fluoride does not cause genetic damage, was made aware that his data showed a dose-dependent increase in chromosome damage in the testes cells of mice drinking as little as one part per million fluoride in their drinking water. Thereafter, he altered his data (which he admitted in court could not be changed because of the blind design of his experiments) as follows in an attempt to cover up the link between fluoride and genetic damage which his very own study showed. Note, in the following table, how in the 'data presented in court' the stepwise increase in fluoride level was accompanied by an increase in genetic damage. Note also how this dose-dependent increase in genetic damage was destroyed in the paper he finally published in *Mutation Research*.

ALTERATION OF DATA BETWEEN
GEORGE MARTIN'S TESTIMONY IN COURT
AND THE SUBSEQUENT PUBLICATION OF HIS DATA
IN *MUTATION RESEARCH*

Fluoride in the Drinking Water	Percent of Testes Cells with Chromosome Damage	
	'Data presented in court'	'Data presented in *Mutation Research*'
0 ppm	0.40%	0.40%
1 ppm	0.65%	1.00%
5 ppm	1.20%	0.40%
10 ppm	3.28%	2.70%

On June 30, 1978, during his testimony, Dr. Martin admitted that the above table showed a dose-dependent increase in chromosomal damage from zero to 10 parts per million. However, he claimed that this step-wise increase was not sustained at higher doses of 50 and 100 parts per million. But since one would expect excessive chromosome damage at higher fluoride concentrations, and since Dr. Martin didn't score excessively damaged cells, referred to as ball metaphase, it was not surprising that he scored zero chromosomal damage at the two highest fluoride concentrations.

The following are excerpts from an article titled 'Is Science Censored?', which appeared in the September 14, 1992 issue of *Newsweek*:

> "'Publicity . . . would certainly follow', fretted the editor of one top journal. 'A possible general panic', predicted a researcher. Both were explaining why a study linking childhood leukemia to fluorescent lights would not be published. That fear trumped the conclusion of other reviewers — scientists who evaluate whether a manuscript should be published in a journal — who called the paper 'intriguing' and an 'extraordinary piece of deductive reasoning.' The paper was rejected.
>
> "A *New England Journal of Medicine* reviewer called it 'an intriguing idea that can be readily tested,'

*but **NEJM** rejected it 'because it does not warrant the publicity.' **The Lancet** feared a 'general panic in which nurseries are plunged into semi-darkness.'*

*"One leading cancer journal [**Journal of the National Cancer Institute**], for instance, recently published an industry [Procter and Gamble] study concluding that the fluoride added to drinking water does not increase the risk of cancer in lab animals. That same journal rejected a government study, by researchers at the National Institute of Environmental Health Sciences [the very scientists from Battelle and the National Institute of Environmental Health Sciences that carried out the fluoride-cancer research mandated by Congress] that reported an increase in rare bone cancers among male rats fed fluoride. The journal explained that it does not publish lab-animal studies anymore. 'No one wants to touch this', says toxicologist James Huff of NIEHS about the persistent evidence that fluoride poses some hazard."*

Chapter 20

Look What They've Done To Our Courts, Mom

"I entered an injunction against the fluoridation of the public water supply for a large portion of Allegheny County, Pennsylvania. I did this after a very lengthy series of hearings on the issue. . . . Prior to my hearing this case, I gave the matter of fluoridation little, if any, thought, but I received quite an education, and noted that the proponents of fluoridation do nothing more than try to impugn the objectivity of those who oppose fluoridation."

John P. Flaherty, Justice
Supreme Court of Pennsylvania

"As a judge who has to run for office every two years, and have since my election in 1948, had to defeat six men lawyers to retain it, I should be by now sufficiently a politician to realize that I may be jeopardizing my office at the next election if I oppose fluoridation, but my conscience does not allow me to remain silent on the issue when I see such ignorance as to the physical effects of fluoride and blind acceptance of it as measure made in Heaven itself for the benefit of our children."

Judge Beatrice J. Brown
Brattleboro, Vermont

The Trial Courts

Upset at the results of the 1977 Congressional Hearings, which merely censured the National Cancer Institute for their cover-up and refusal to supply the cancer data requested by Congressman James Delaney and Burk and Yiamouyiannis, opponents of fluoridation went to the courts with the following results.

Nov. 6, 1978: Despite testimony from profluoridationists such as Dr. George Martin of the National Institute of Dental Research, Dr. Leo Kinlen from the Royal College of Physicians, Dr. D. J. Newell, from the Royal Statistical Society, Dr. Donald Taves from the National Academy of Sciences, and Dr. Marvin Schneiderman from the National Cancer Institute — Judge John P. Flaherty, also chairman of the Pennsylvania Academy of Sciences, ruled that he was *"compellingly convinced"* that fluoride is a carcinogen and ordered a halt to fluoridation. In his decision, he stated: *"Point by point, every criticism made of the B-Y [Burk-Yiamouyiannis] Study was met and explained"*.[28]

Feb. 22, 1982: In Texas, after 11 days of hearings, Judge Anthony J.P. Farris ruled that *"Plaintiffs had the burden to introduce overwhelming evidence in this case"* that fluoridation was unsafe and ineffective and that they *"have not overcome their enormous burden"* and denied the petition to stop fluoridation. In subsequently (5/24/82) issuing findings of fact in this case, he did state that *"The considerable amount of evidence introduced, heard and considered by this court . . . shows . . . that the artificial fluoridation of water supplies . . . may cause or contribute to the cause of cancer, genetic damage, intolerant reactions, and chronic toxicity, including dental mottling, in man; that the said artificial fluoridation may aggravate malnutrition and existing illnesses in man; and that the value of said artificial fluoridation is in some doubt as to the reduction of tooth decay in man."*

Feb. 28, 1982: In Illinois, after 40 days of hearings devoted primarily to testimony regarding fluoridation and cancer, Judge Ronald Niemann ruled *"A conclusion that fluoridation is a safe and effective means of promoting dental health cannot be supported by this record"* and ordered a halt to fluoridation.

---

[28] Apparently, John Small, who attended the case, felt that the case was not going too well and, along with his cronies, including Stephen Barrett, Robert Hoover, and others, worked with Consumers Union to publish an article to attack witnesses in the Pittsburgh case who were testifying against fluoridation. It was introduced on one of the last days of the case (July 19, 1978) to impugn the integrity of these witnesses, but to the chagrin of Small and his conspirators, was disregarded by the court.

Nov. 23, 1982: In South Carolina, after 9 days of hearings, Master in Equity Louis E. Condon ruled that *"To believe the Plaintiffs, one must believe that the entire established medical and scientific community of this Country and other foreign countries which have studied the subject had conspired to promote fluoridation and cover up its hazards. Such a conspiracy is improbable and has not been proven in this case. Fluoride regulated at one part per million in the drinking water of the city of Charleston has not been shown to constitute a health hazard or a public nuisance . . . the Plaintiffs have failed to meet their burden of proof and, therefore, the Plaintiff's Complaint requesting injunctive relief must be and is denied."*

The Appeals Courts

Even the Pennsylvania Supreme Court, after fluoridation had been proven harmful in its lower court, ruled that, nonetheless, the court did not have the power to intervene in behalf of the health and safety of its citizens.

In 1982, after 40 days of testimony, the Illinois trial court determined that fluoridation of public water supplies created a public health hazard and determined that the Illinois mandatory fluoridation law was unconstitutional, and ordered a halt to it. In Alton, Illinois, in his decision, the presiding Judge Ronald Niemann said:

"Considering the part of the plaintiffs' case that is credible, together with the failure of the State to adequately explain the scope of the risks to the public the Court orders an injunction to issue against the Department of Public Health, the Environmental Protection Agency and to the Alton Water Company from further use of artificial fluoride in the public water supply.

"This record is barren of any credible and reputable, scientific epidemiological studies and / or analysis of statistical data which would support the Illinois Legislature's determination that fluoridation of public water supplies is both a safe and effective means of promoting public health.

"The legislation that exposes the public to the risk, uncertain in its scope, of unhealthy side effects of artificial fluoridation of the public water supply is __unreasonable__ and a violation of the

due process clause of the Illinois Constitution of 1970" (emphasis added).

In overturning Judge Niemann's order, the Illinois Supreme Court stated: *"We construe the circuit court's comment to mean that plaintiffs have shown, not that the risk was so great that fluoridation was unreasonable, but that the question was shown to be debatable."*

They Wouldn't Even Listen

The very courts themselves seem to be intimidated by the fluoridation issue. Local courts in New York City, New York; Kansas City, Missouri; Houston, Texas; Clinton, Indiana; and Cincinnati, Ohio as well as the Federal District Court in Cleveland, Ohio have refused to even hear or act on the cases, despite the fact that fluoridation had already been proven harmful in other courts. The argument in all these cases can basically be summarized by the judgement of the U.S. Sixth Circuit Court of Appeals, which held, in effect, that the state has the power to add a substance to the public water supply that causes ill-health or death without violating the rights of the citizens — even if the addition is made for no good reason whatsoever — and that therefore the only relief that citizens can obtain is legislative relief.

Why haven't **Consumer Reports**, Stephen Barrett and others who issue false and defamatory statements been sued for libel and slander? Why haven't bureaucrats responsible for illegally spending tax monies to influence elections been prosecuted and sent to jail? Why haven't bureaucrats who have lied in court while under oath been prosecuted for perjury?

In many cases they have. However, when legal action was taken against **Consumer Reports**, the court didn't even allow a hearing on the case. The court claimed **Consumer Reports'** right to freedom of speech outweighed the plaintiffs right to due process of the law.

When charges concerning Dr. Schneiderman's alleged perjury in the Pittsburgh court case were brought before the district attorney's office, they pointed out it would be virtually impossible to convict anyone on perjury and they rarely, if ever, prosecute such cases.

Chapter 21

Good News

"Noted Stephen J. Marx, M.D., with the National Institute of Arthritis, Diabetes, and Digestive and Kidney Diseases: . . . 'If we were just handling this as an environmental contaminant, we could . . . recommend that it (fluoride) be kept below half a part per million (0.5 mg/l)'"

Medical Tribune, April 20, 1989

"Bill Hirzy, president of the Environmental Protection Agency's National Federation of Federal Employees . . . said yesterday, 'the EPA has been endorsing water fluoridation for prevention of tooth decay. But based on our statisticians' review of Mr. Yiamouyiannis' findings, we feel it's time to suspend that support.'"

Washington Times, May 1, 1989

"Yiamouyiannis compared decay rates in terms of decayed, missing, and filled permanent teeth. The average decay rates for all the children aged five to 17 were 2.0 teeth for both fluoridated and nonfluoridated areas . . . Janet A. Brunelle, a statistician in the epidemiology program at NIDR, tells C & EN the[ir] results for teeth 'are in a box somewhere' and she does not remember exactly what they are."

Chemical & Engineering News, May 8, 1989

"[S]ome experts argue that the risks [of fluoridation] outweigh the benefits, and the practice should be stopped . . . Few studies of dental fluorosis have been performed in Britain, but . . . as soon as they look for it they find it to be widespread."

London Sunday Times, May 28, 1989

"A lot of responsible scientists question the value of fluoridation."
Columbia Journalism Review, May/June 1989

"Yiamouyiannis . . . compared the number of decayed, missing and filled teeth among children in an area with fluoridation, without fluoridation, and with partial fluoridation. He found no statistically significant differences among children of any age group."

Boston Globe, June 19, 1989

"Shelves of studies . . . have asked the questions, does fluoride cripple the bones, discolor the teeth, cause birth defects and cancer? The resounding answer has been, who knows ?"

Jack Anderson, Syndicated Columnist, June 24, 1989

"Now, liberal legislators, an environmental advocacy group, a respected chemical trade journal and even scientists at the U.S. Environmental Protection Agency are challenging the conventional wisdom of fluoride's necessity and safety."

Pittsburgh Press, July 23, 1988

"Armed with decades of evidence, including a surprising drop in cavity rates in countries that have never fluoridated their water, scientists are asking: Does fluoride in drinking water effectively reduce cavities? Or does it instead contaminate water in ways that it may be upping cancer cases, skeletal disorders, birth defects — and even tooth erosion?"

Longevity, July 1989

"On Aug 28 William L. Marcus, chief toxicologist for the Environmental Protection Agency's drinking water programme, claimed that the original findings of the NTP study showed the cancer hazard from fluoridated drinking water to be greater than the NTP was telling the public . . . The Battelle study's principal finding was the occurrence of an extremely rare liver cancer, hepatochalongiocarcinoma, in male and female mice . . . Dr. Marcus believes the Battelle diagnosis of liver cancers was sound and should have been included in the NTP report. This, he says, would change 'the (NTP) equivocal finding . . . to at least some evidence or clear evidence of carcinogenicity.'"

The Lancet, September 22, 1990

*"The Environmental Protection Agency has been ordered to
reinstate a senior scientist [William Marcus] and pay him
$50,000 for emotional distress after he was fired for what he
claimed were his whistle-blowing activities, his lawyer said
yesterday. In ordering Marcus's reinstatement, administrative
law judge David Clarke Jr . . . concluded the reasons given for
the firing were 'a pretext' and that he really was dismissed
'because he publicly questioned and opposed EPA's fluoride
policy.'"*
Washington Post, December 9, 1992

The good news is that the bandwagon to promote fluoridation is
falling apart. Prestigious organizations such as the American
Chemical Society are now publishing significant articles questioning the safety and effectiveness of fluoride. For example, the
August 1, 1988 issue of ***Chemical and Engineering News***
published a 17-page cover article on fluoridation and the attempts of fluoridation promoters to suppress the publication of
articles which might even indicate that fluoridation is unsafe or
ineffective.

Defections of former promoters of fluoridation even when
they are punished as a result leave fluoridation promoters
wondering *"Is there something we can't buy?"*

Yes. For example, John Colquhoun.

In 1980, Dr. John Colquhoun was the principle dental officer
of Auckland, New Zealand and Chairman of the Fluoridation
Promotion Committee of the New Zealand Dental Health Foundation. On his return from a world-wide tour to gather information regarding fluoride and fluoridation, he decided to examine
tooth decay records of all 12- and 13-year-old schoolchildren in
New Zealand. He found that there was no difference in tooth
decay rates in children living in fluoridated and nonfluoridated
areas. Furthermore, he found that within fluoridated areas, a
substantial number of the children had dental fluorosis. When
he decided to make this news public, his superiors in the health
department threatened him with the loss of his job and/or
retirement benefits. The good news is that he made the informa-

tion public anyhow, even though he was forced into early retirement with a reduced pension as a result.

In December 1973, as a special consultant to the health minister of British Columbia, Dr. Richard Foulkes authored a report recommending mandatory fluoridation for the province. But after reviewing the evidence in 1992, he has concluded that *"fluoridation of community water supplies can no longer be held to be safe or effective in the reduction of tooth decay . . . Even in 1973, we should have known this was a dangerous chemical."* He points out that when he originally did his report, the information given to him was biased and selected. Having seen both sides, he has now recommended a halt to all fluoridation.

In 1992, Michael Perrone, a legislative assistant in New Jersey, contacted the Food and Drug Administration (FDA) requesting all the information they had in their files regarding the safety and effectiveness of fluoride tablets and drops. After hounding them for six months, the FDA admitted that they had nothing to show that fluoride tablets or drops were either safe or effective in reducing tooth decay. They have since informed Perrone that because of this lack of data, the FDA will probably have to pull fluoride tablets and drops off the market. [Hopefully this will have occurred by the time this book is published].

In the midst of doing his research on fluoridation and tooth decay in 1989, Dr. Yiamouyiannis had the occasion to contact Dr. Anthony Volpe, world-wide dental director for Colgate-Palmolive, the world's largest manufacturer of toothpaste. During the conversation, Dr. Yiamouyiannis told Dr. Volpe about the results of his 40,000 schoolchildren dental survey with regard to fluoridation of public water supplies. Dr. Volpe admitted that he never did believe that fluoridation of public water supplies could be or was effective in reducing tooth decay.

At the 1992 Society of Toxicology meeting, Dr. James Huff of the U.S. National Institute of Environmental Health Sciences stated unequivocally that U.S. National Toxicology Program two-year rodent study *"found a rare bone cancer called osteosarcoma in fluoride-exposed male rats."* Huff also said he believes *"that the reason these animals got a few osteosarcomas of the bone was because they were given fluoride."* According to

Stan Freni of the FDA, the scientists at the National Institute of Environmental Health Sciences are convinced that fluoride causes bone cancer.

Scientists at the Environmental Protection Agency are striking out hard against the crooked higher-level bureaucrats at the USEPA. Dr. William Marcus, who refused to play along with the USEPA's attempted cover-up of fluoride hazards, was fired. Dr. Marcus came right back and sued the USEPA — and won. The USEPA's union, while pleased with the judge's decision to reinstate Dr. Marcus, wanted the court to take further action and commented:

"Judge Clarke took particular notice of the Inspector General's Office's shredding of evidentiary notes, contrary to law and regulation. He unfortunately did not mention witness tampering by management (one witness said that he had been threatened with dire consequences if gave testimony which helped Dr. Marcus's case) nor what appear to be, based on testimony by a knowledgeable labor lawyer, management forgeries of time cards used to entrap Dr. Marcus. Justice is now half done. Now those management officials who lied, conspired and exercised power arrogantly to cause pain and temporary humiliation to Dr. Marcus, a huge work load for the Union, and embarrassment and expense to the Agency must be shown the same door that Dr. Marcus was shown in May.

"These officials include Inspector General John Martin and his staffer Francis Kiley, Margaret Stasikowski, Dr. Marcus's supervisor in the Criteria and Standards Division, and Tudor Davies, Directory of the Office of Science and Technology and the man who fired Dr. Marcus. These people were the chief instrumentalities of the conspiracy against Dr. Marcus within EPA."

According to the latest information, most of the advanced Western European countries have banned fluoridation or given it up. Belgium, West Germany, and Sweden have abandoned their pilot fluoridation experiments on human populations and are not fluoridating any public water supplies. Sweden, Denmark, and Holland have banned it outright. Many other countries, such as France, Italy, and Norway, have never fluoridated their drinking water. Only about 2% of the total population of

Europe is living in a fluoridated area.

Groups formerly supporting fluoridation are now retracting their endorsements. For example, the National PTA has withdrawn its endorsement of fluoridation of public water supplies. Some of its affiliates have gone even further and have come out against fluoride programs.

Chapter 22

The Solution

You are the solution. You can make this happen. The major sacrifices have been made and, as of June 1993, we have them on the run. If you want to do something about it, you can help by making regular contributions to the Safe Water Foundation until we stop fluoridation — the sooner the better. You can purchase copies of this book and sell them to those around you who are interested. I would advise you to sell them — not give them away — for two reasons: people are far more likely to read books they buy rather than books that they are given and having them purchase the book gets them involved.

Book orders and donations can be sent to:

Safe Water Foundation
6439 Taggart Road
Delaware, Ohio 43015

Upon receiving your donation, we can put you in the network and get you together with others in your area. Get your own recruits. This is a matter of your health and the health of your loved ones. It's a matter of taking back the control of your government.

In short, the ultimate solution to the fluoride problem is to have it removed from public water systems around the country. And you can stop it through the political process if you work hard enough and soon enough.

Remember, the reason things have gotten so bad is because citizens have ignored their responsibility to participate in politics and government. Apathy among the citizens has led to apathetic politicians who have turned over their functions to the bureaucrats. Bureaucrats entrusted to safeguard the health of Americans are not doing their job; worse yet, in an attempt to stabilize themselves in their 'do nothing' jobs, they have allied themselves with those industries which they were originally created to regulate. In the case of fluoridation, they have gone one step further and promoted a measure which has now been proven harmful. Who can protect us from our 'protectors'? You!

The reason bureaucrats have become so fanatic and sloppy in their promotion of fluoridation is because they realize that fluoride can become the catalyst that the people can rally behind to destroy their pork barrel and power base. By showing that fluoridation is a fraud, you can help give the public their first good look at the corruption and incompetence of the unelected bureaucrats that run our government and their collusion with vested interests.

In the meantime . . .

If you live in a fluoridated area, most of the fluoride you ingest can be removed from your diet by purchasing distilled water at the supermarket, by having distilled water delivered to your home, or by purchasing a home water distiller.

The home distiller is the best method and also the best way to get distilled water. It is the only reliable home water purification system for taking fluoride out of the water. The device you buy should produce at least 1 gallon per day per family member. It should contain a holding tank of 2-3 gallons or more. It should be automatic with an automatic water feed and an automatic turnoff when the holding tank is full. It should be designed so that after the water is distilled, the only material the water comes in contact with is stainless steel or glass. Try to avoid water distillers that have a plastic holding tank.

I recommend the following two distillers as being, in my experience, as good as or better than other water purifiers on the market. For tabletop models, the Durastill model 30J with a CT 4.0 holding tank, price about $900 (for information contact Durastill, 4200 Northeast Birmingham Road, Kansas City, Missouri 64117); for floor models, the Aqua D 2000 with a 10 gallon holding tank by Pure Water, Inc., price about $1400 (for information, contact Pure Water, Inc., Box 83226, Lincoln Nebraska 68501). Pure Water Inc. also has the Aqua D 2000 Plus, price about $1500, which reduces or eliminates the need to even clean out the boiling chamber.

The next most convenient method is having distilled water delivered to your home. Make sure what is delivered is distilled water with no additives. There are some companies that sell 'purified' water that is more harmful than the water you are getting out of your tap. The problems with home delivery are the inconvenience of having to lift 5-gallon bottles of water, the clutter of 5-gallon bottles lying around from one delivery to the next, and the lower quality of the water if the local water suppliers only deliver the water in plastic containers.

The least convenient method is purchasing water at your local supermarket, grocery store, health food store, etc. and having to lug bottles of water back home. Again, I recommend that you get distilled water. If you decide to get another type of bottled water, check with the water supplier to determine the fluoride content. Ideally, the fluoride content should be two-tenths part per million or less.

For single people buying water at retail stores may be reasonable, but for larger families, it is a bothersome chore. In addition, distilled water purchased at these retail stores is almost invariably sold in plastic containers.

Fluoride-free or at least low-fluoride water should be used for drinking as well as for the cooking and preparation of all food and drinks. For more information on this and how to avoid fluoride while away from home, see Chapter 12.

Appendix

Chapter 1 Speeding Up the Aging Process

"The Village Where People are Old before their Time", *Stern*, Volume 30, pp. 107-108, 111-112 (1978).

G. Frada, et al., "On the Behavior of Thyroid Function in Subjects with Hydrofluorosis in an Endemic Center in Sicily", *Minerva Medica*, Volume 60, pp. 545-549 (1969).

"Relief Elusive As Life is Crippled." *The Hindu*, January 24, 1982.

S.S. Jolly, et al., "Endemic Fluorosis in Punjab I. Skeletal Aspect", *Fluoride*, Volume 6, pp. 4-18 (1973).

G.V. Black and Frederic McKay, "Mottled Teeth: An Endemic Developmental Imperfection of the Enamel Heretofore Unknown in the Literature of Dentistry", *Dental Cosmos*, Volume 58, No. 2, pp. 129-156 (1916).

Steven Jacobsen, et al., "Regional Variation in the Incidence of Hip Fracture", *Journal of the American Medical Association*, Volume 264, pp. 500-502 (1990).

Nicholas Leone, et al., "Medical Aspects of Excessive Fluoride in a Water Supply", *Public Health Reports*, Volume 69, pp. 925-936 (1954).

J. David Erickson, "Mortality of Selected Cities with Fluoridated and Non-fluoridated Water Supplies", *New England Journal of Medicine*, Volume 298, pp. 1112-1116 (1978).

John Yiamouyiannis, unpublished report (1983).

E.R. Schlesinger et al., "Newburgh-Kingston caries-fluorine study. XIII. Pediatric findings after ten years", *Journal of the American Dental Association*, Volume 52, pp. 296-306 (1956).

J. Caffey, "On fibrous defects in cortical walls: their radiologic appearance, structure, prevalence, natural course, and diagnostic significance", *Advances in Pediatrics*, S.V. Levin, editor; 1955, pp. 13-51.

Chapter 2 Signs of Fluoride Poisoning in the Western World

"1983 USPDI-Drug Informational for the Health Care Provider", *United States Pharmacopeial Convention*, Volume I, pp. 805-807 (1982).

"1983 USPDI-Drug Informational for the Health Care Provider", *United States Pharmacopeial Convention*, Volume II, pp. 656-657 (1982).

1991 Physicians' Desk Reference, Medical Economics Company 1983, pp. 1976-1977.

Kathy Krausfelder, Letter to Wini Silko, January 4, 1993.

William Murphy, Letter to George Waldbott, May 4, 1965.

John Shea, et al., "Allergy to Fluoride", *Annals of Allergy*, Volume 25, pp. 388-391 (1967).

G.W. Grimbergen, "A Double-Blind Test for Determination of Intolerance to Fluoridated Water", *Fluoride*, Volume 7, pp 146-152 (1974).

Jonathan Forman, "What Looks Like a Neurosis May be a Fluorosis", *Clinical Physiology*, pp. 245-251 (Winter 1963).

Luis Juncos and James Donadio, "Renal Failure and Fluorosis", *Journal of the American Medical Association*, Volume 222, pp. 783-785 (1972).

Sohan Manocha, et al., "Cytochemical Response of Kidney, Liver and Nervous System to Fluoride Ions in Drinking Water", *Histochemical Journal*, Volume 7, pp. 343-355 (1975).

William Ramseyer, et al., "Effect of Sodium Fluoride Administration on Body Changes in Old Rats", *Journal of Gerontology*, Volume 12, No. 14, pp. 14-19 (1957).

George Waldbott, "Fluoridation: A Clinician's Experience", *Southern Medical Journal*, Volume 73, No. 3, pp. 301-306 (1980).

Bertram Carnow and Shirley Conibear, "Case Study of the Effects of Aluminum Smelting on the Health of Alcan Workers in Kitimat", British Columbia, Canada, 1977, 40 pp.

V. Soyseth and J. Kongerud, "Prevalence of respiratory disorders among aluminium potroom workers in relation to exposure to fluoride", *Br J Ind Med*, Volume 49, pp. 125-30 (1992).

V. N. Medvedeva, "The diagnosis and treatment of osteoarthrosis deformans in subjects in contact with fluorine compounds", *Vrach-Delo.*, Issue 8, pp. 76-78 (1992).

M. Klotz, "Strange Case of Periostitis Hyperplastica of Undetermined Etiology (Fluorine Injury) in an Infant", *Arch. Kinderheilkd.*, Volume 117, pp. 267-271 (1939).

M. M. Murray and D. C. Wilson, "Fluorine Hazards with Special Reference to Some Social Consequence of Industrial Processes", *Lancet* , Volume 2, pp. 821-824 (1946).

K. Roholm, *Fluorine Intoxication: A Clinical-Hygenic Study*, 1937.

E. Speder, "Generalized Osteopetrosis or 'Marble Skeleton' is not a Rate Disease: Its frequency in Fluoride Poisoning", *Journal Radiol, Electrol.*, Volume 20, pp. 1-11 (1936).

H. H. Schlegel, "Industrial Skeletal Fluorosis: A Brief Report on 60 Cases from Aluminum Foundries", *Soz. Praeventivmed.*, Volume 19, pp. 269-274 (1974).

J. Franke, "Histological Changes of Human Fluorosis, Experimental Fluorosis in Animals and Osteoporosis Following Sodium Fluoride therapy", *Fluoride*, Volume 5, pp. 182-199 (1972).

P. Sadtler, "Fluorine Gases in atmosphere as Industrial Waste Blamed for Death and Chronic Poisoning of Donora and Webster, Pennsylvania Inhabitants", *Chemical and Engineering News*, Volume 26, pp. 3692 (1948).

K. Roholm, "The Fog Disaster in the Meuse Valley: A Fluorine Intoxication", *Journal of Industrial Hygiene and Toxicology*, Volume 19, pp. 126-137 (1937).

Williams & Wilkins,*Clinical Toxicology of Commercial Products*, pp. II-4, II-112, II-129, II-138 (1984).

Environmental Action, pp. 18, July/August 1984.

Yngve Ericsson and Britta Forsman, "Fluoride retained from mouthrinses and dentifrices in preschool children", *Caries Research*, Volume 3, pp. 290-299 (1969).

John Yiamouyiannis, unpublished report, 1979.

W. L. Augenstein, et al., "Fluoride ingestion in children: a review of 87 cases", *Pediatrics*, Volume 88, pp. 907-912 (1991).

G. Konstantinidis, et al., "Drug poisoning in children in Vojvodina", *Arh Hig Rada Toksikol* , Volume 42, pp. 391-396 (1991).

R. Anderson, et al., "Fluoride Intoxication in a Dialysis Unit—Maryland", *Morbidity and Mortality Weekly Report*, Volume 29, pp. 134-136 (1980).

Charles Wax, "Field Investigation Report", State of Maryland Department of Health and Mental Hygiene, March 19, 1980, 67 pp.

George Waldbott, "Mass Intoxication from Accidental Over-Fluoridation of Drinking Water", *Clinical Toxicology*, Volume 18, No. 5, pp. 531-541 (1981).

[Listed below are additional cases of mass fluoride poisoning due to fluoride spills:

Robert Clarke, et al., "Acute Fluoride Poisoning—North Carolina", *Morbidity and Mortality Weekly Report*, Volume 23, pp. 199 (1974).

Richard Hoffman, et al., "Acute Fluoride Poisoning in a New Mexico Elementary School", *Pediatrics*, Volume 65, No. 5, pp. 897-900 (1980).

Kenneth Powell, et al., "Fluoride Poisoning in Michigan—For Administrative Use—Limited Distribution—Not for Publication", *U.S. Public Health Service, Center for Disease Control-Atlanta*, EPI 78-24-2, pp. 12, (1978)

Fluoride Spill in Marin County California, reported in the November 25, 1977 issue of the *San Rafael (California) Independent Journal*.

Fluoride Spill in Jonesboro, Maine, reported in the October 19, 1981 issue of *The Maine Paper*, p.3.

Fluoride Spill in Potsdam, New York, report in the August 18, 1981 issue of the *Potsdam (New York) Courier-Freeman*.

L. R. Petersen, et al, "Community Health Effects of a Municipal Water Supply Hyperfluoridation Accident", *American Journal of Public Health*, Volume 78, pages 711-713 (1988).

Brad Gessner, et al., *Hooper Bay Water-borne Outbreak: Interim Report #1*, Dept of Health and Social Services of Alaska, June 11, 1992

"Statement on Water Treatment Program", *Antigo Daily Journal*, April 24, 1989, page 10.

Mike Mathes, "Failsafe?", *Kiel (Wisconsin) Tri-County Record*, October 26, 1990, p. 4.

[The most frightening aspect of this list is that such spills have occurred in other places and are probably occurring in every fluoridated area but are not being reported. Attempts were made to cover up the Annapolis and Marin County spills. People in Annapolis were not told about the spill until two weeks after it occurred, and only then when the local newspaper leaked the news. As an excuse, the county "health" officer stated: "We did not want to jeopardize the fluoridation program." In Marin County, people were not notified of the spill until one week later.]

Norm Hartman, "State Health Director Warns of Contaminated Niagara Brand Drinking Water", *California Department of Health Services*, March 30, 1989.

Taped interview with Ms. Terry Leder on October 29, 1979.

Naham C. Cons, et al, "Albany Topical Fluoride Study", *Journal of the American Dental Association*, Volume 80, pp. 777-781 (1970).

Herschel S. Horowitz and Helen S. Lucye, "A Clinical Study of Stannous Fluoride in a Prophylaxis Paste and as a Solution", *Journal of Oral Therapeutics and Pharmacology*, Volume 3, pp. 17-25 (1967).

"Continuing Evaluation of the Use of Fluorides", *American Association for the Advancement of Science*, Washington, D.C., p. 20 (1979).

Orville J. Stone and Carolyn J. Willis, "The Effect of Stannous Fluoride and Stannous Chloride on Inflammation", *Toxicology and Applied Pharmacology*, Volume 13, pp. 332-338 (1968).

J. Lindle, et al., "The Effect of Topical Application of Fluorides on the Gingival Tissues", *Journal of Periodontal Research*, Volume 6, pp. 211-217 (1971).

L. K. Rubenstein and M. A. Avent, "Frequency of undesirable side-effects following professionally applied topical fluoride", *ASDC J. Dent. Child.*, Volume 54, pp. 245-247 (1987).

Milton A. Saunders, "Fluoride Toothpastes: A Cause of Acne-Like Eruptions", *Archives of Dermatology*, Volume 111, p. 793 (1975).

J. Ramsey Mellette, et al., "Fluoride Toothpaste: A Cause of Perioral Dermatitis", *Archives of Dermatology*, Volume 112, pp. 730-731 (1976).

Merck Index, Merck and Company, Inc., Rahway, New Jersey, 1968, p. 959.

[Other studies showing that fluoridated water depresses thyroid activity are listed below:

Viktor Gorlitzer Von Mundy, "Influence of Fluorine and Iodine on the Metabolism, Particularly on the Thyroid Gland", *Muenchener Medicische Wochenschrift*, Volume 105, pp. 182-186 (1963).

A. Benagiano, "The Effect of Sodium Fluoride on Thyroid Enzymes and Basal Metabolism the Rat", *Annali Di Stomatologia*, Volume 14, pp. 601-619 (1965).

A. Jentzer, "The Effect of Sodium Fluoride on Thyroid Enzymes and Basal Metabolism in the Rat", *Schweize Medizinishe Wochschrift*, Volume 85, pp. 663-664 (1955).

E. Domzalska, "Influence of Sodium Fluoride on Hypophysis, Thyroid Gland, Parathyroid, and Adrenal Gland in the White Rat", *Czas. Stomat.*, Volume 19, pp. 132-145 (1966).

G. Ritzel, "Thyroxine Metabolism and Fluoridation Water", *Internationale Zeitschrift fur Vitaminforschung*, Volume 34, No. 4, pp. 422-426 (1964).

A.J. Held, "Fluoride and the Thyroid Gland", *Bull. Acad. Suisse Sci. Med.*, Volume 9, pp. 132-145 (1953).

A. Benagiano and S. Firoentini, "Experimental Investigation of the Pharmacological Action of Fluoride", *ORCA. Proceedings of the 6th Congress of the European Organization for Research on Fluorine and Dental Caries Prevention*, University of Pavia, Italy (1959).

T. Burkov, "Changes in the C14-Carbonate Uptake in Mineralized Tissues and of Radioiodine in the Thyroid Gland of the Rat Under the Influence of Sodium Fluoride", *Stomatologiya*, Volume 47, pp. 1-5 (1968).

Fung-Chang Sung, et al., "Studies of the Effect of Salt Iodization on Endemic Goiter in Taiwan", *Journal of Formosan Medical Association*, Volume 72, pp. 96-103 (1973).

V. Stolc and J. Podoba, "Effect of Fluoride on the Biogenesis of Thyroid Hormones", *Nature*, Volume 188, No. 4753, pp. 855-856 (1960).

Pierre-M. Galleti and Gustave Joyet, "Effect of Fluorine of Thyroidal Iodine Metabolism in Hyperthyroidism", *Journal of Clinical Endocrinology and Metabolism*, Volume 18, pp. 1102-1110 (1958).

Donald Hillman, et al., "Hypothyroidism and Anemia Related to Fluoride in Dairy Cattle", *Journal of Dairy Science*, Volume 62, No. 3, pp. 416-423 (1979).]

Richard DeSwarte, "Drug Allergy", *Allergic Diseases, Diagnosis and Management*, J.B. Lippincott Co., Philadelphia, 1980, pp. 452-507.

[The following is a partial list of laboratory studies showing that low levels of fluoride in water has a disruptive effect on various tissues.

G. Borsotti and S. Frugis, "Morphologic Studies of Fluorotic Kidneys and Livers of Experimental Animals", *Rassegna Internazionale di Stomatologia Pratica*, Volume 14, No. 1, pp. 21-30 (1963).

Vilber A. O. Bello and Hillel J. Gitelman, "High Fluoride Exposure in Hemodialysis Patients", *American Journal of Kidney Diseases*, Volume 15: 320-324 (1990).

T. Takamori, "The Heart Changes of Growing Albino Rats Fed on Varied Contents of Fluorine", *The Toxicology of Fluorine, Symposium*, Bern, October 1962 pp. 125-129.

C. Faenzi, "Vascular and Parenchymal Lesions by Fluoride Associated with High Lipid Diet", *Annali di Stomatologia*, Volume 10, No. 9, pp. 807-822 (1961).

G. Borsotti, "Effects of Fluoride on Experimental Animals", *Rassegna Internazionale di Stomatologia Practica*, Volume 12, pp. 45-71 (1962).

A.F. Aksyuk and G.V. Gulychev, "Physiological Effects of Small Amounts of Fluoride on the Organism", *Gigiena i Sanitariya*, Volume 27, No. 12, pp. 7-10 (1962).

C. Faenzi, "Devitaminizing Action of Waters at Low Fluorine Content. II. Sodium Fluoride and Lesions by Thiamine Deficiency", *Annali di Stomatologia*, Volume 12, pp. 965-975 (1963).

T. Burkov and T. Burkova, "Early Morphological and Some Enzymochemical Changes in the Liver and Oral Mucosa Under the Effect of Fluoride-Containing Mineral Waters", *Nauchno-Izledovatelskiya Stomatologichen Institut.*, Volume 12, pp. 1-9 (1969).

R.D. Gabovich, et al., "Histochemical and Biochemical Changes in the Liver of Experimental Animals During Prolonged Use of Water with Varying Fluorine Levels", *Gig. Naselen. Mest. Resp. Mezhved. Sb.*, Volume 9, pp. 102-107 (1970).

Y. Yoshida, "Experimental Studies on Chronic Fluorine Poisoning", *Japanese Journal of Industrial Health*, Volume 1, pp. 683-690 (1959).]

[The following is a list of some additional clinical studies on fluoride-induced diseases.

H. Odenthal and H.L. Wieneke, "Chronic Fluorine Poisoning and Osteomyelosclerosis", *Deutsche Medizinische Wochenschrift*, Volume 84, pp. 725-728 (1959).

G. Frada, "Research on Endemic Fluorosis", *Minerva Medica*, Volume 54, pp. 45-59 (1963).

Amarjit Singh, "Endemic Fluorosis", *The Toxicology of Fluorine, Symposium, Bern, Basel, Schwabe and Co.*, pp. 49-52 (1964).

Dopuw Steyn, "Chronic Fluorine Poisoning Caused by Drinking of Subterranean Waters Containing Excessive Quantities of Flourine", *The Toxicology of Fluorine Symposium, Bern, Basel, Schwabe and Co.*, pp. 53-57 (1964).

M.G. Geall and L.J. Beilin, "Sodium Fluoride and Optic Neuritis", *British Medical Journal*, Volume II, pp. 355-356 (1964).

V.R. Ovechkin, "Involvement of the Peripheral Nervous System in Chronic Fluorosis", *Gigiena Truda i Professional'nye Zabolevaniya*, Volume 10, no. 4, p. 87 (1966).

M. M. Webb-Peploe and W. G. Bradley, "Endemic Fluorosis with Neurological Complications in a Hampshire Man", *Journal of Neurology, Neurosurgery and Psychiatry*, Volume 29, pp. 577-583 (1966).

Lawrence G. Blasic and Steven K. Spencer, "Fluoroderma", *Archives of Dermatology*, Volume 115, pp. 1334-1335 (1979).

Michael McIvor, et al., "Hyperkalemia and Cardiac Arrest from Fluoride Exposure during Hemodialysis", *American Journal of Cardiology*, Volume 51, pp. 901-902 (1983).

C. Williams, et al., "Bone Fluoride in Renal Osteodystrophy", *Canadian Society of Nephrology*, 14th Annual Meeting (1981).

A. Rigalli, et al., "Inhibitory Effect of Fluoride on the Secretion of Insulin", *Calcif. Tissue Int.*, Volume 46, pp. 333-338.]

Chapter 3 Disarming the Immune System

John Emsley, et al., "An Unexpectedly Strong Hydrogen Bond: ab Initio Calculations and Spectroscopic Studies of Amide-Fluoride Systems", *Journal of the American Chemical Society*, Volume 103, pp. 24-28 (1981).

Steven L. Edwards, et al., "The Crystal Structure of Fluoride-inhibited Cytochrome c Peroxidase", *Journal of Biological Chemistry*, Volume 259, pp. 12984-12988 (1984).

H. C. Froede and I. B. Wilson, "The Slow Rate of inhibition of Acetylchloinesterase by Fluoride", *Molecular Pharmacology*, Volume 27, pp. 630-633 (1985).

Sheila Gibson, "Effects of Fluoride on Immune System Function", *Complementary Medical Research*, Volume 6, pp. 111-113 (1992)

Peter Wilkinson, "Inhibition of the Immune System with Low Levels of Fluoride (Percentage Inhibition with Chemotactic Response Assay)", Testimony before the Scottish High Court in Edinburgh in the *Case of McColl vs. Strathclyde Regional Council*, pp. 17723-18150, 19328-19492, and Exhibit 636, 1982.

D. W. Allmann and M. Benac, "Effect of Inorganic Fluoride Salts on Urine and Tissue 3'5' Cyclic-AMP Concentration in Vivo", *Journal of Dental Research*, Volume 55 (Supplement B), p. 523 (1976).

H. S. Kleiner and D. W. Allman, "The Effects of Fluoridated Water on Rate Urine and Tissue cAMP Levels", *Archive of Oral Biology*, Volume 27, pp. 107-112 (1982).

S. Jaouni and D. W. Allmann, "Effect of Sodium Fluoride and Aluminum on cAMP, Adenylate Cyclase and Phosphodiesterase Activity", *Journal of Dental Research*, Volume 64, p. 201 (1985).

Israel Rivkin and Elmer L. Becker, "Possible Implication of Cyclic 3'5' - Adenosine Monophosphate in the Chemotaxis of Rabbit Peritoneal Polymorphonuclear Leukocytes", *Federation Proceedings*, Volume 31, p. 2492 (1972).

R. D. Estensen, et al., "Cyclic GMP and Cell Movement", *Nature*, Volume 245, pp. 458-460 (1973).

Gerald Weissmann, et al., "Leukocytic Proteases and the Immunologic Release of Lysomal Enzymes", *American Journal of Pathology*, Volume 68, pp. 539-559 (1972).

J. Gabrovsek, "The Role of the Host in Dental Caries Infection", *Hexagon (Roche)*, Volume 3, No. 3, pp. 17-24 (1980).

Frederick Bloomfield and Marjorie Young, "Influence of Lithium and Fluoride on Degranulation from Human Neutrophils in Vitro", *Inflammation*, Volume 6, No. 3, pp. 257-267 (1982).

Robert A. Clark, "Neutrophil Iodination Reaction Induced by Fluoride: Implications for Degranulation and Metabolic Activation," *Blood*, Volume 57, pp. 913-921 (1981).

W. L. Gabler and P. A. Leong, "Fluoride Inhibition of Polymorphonuclear Leukocytes", *Journal of Dental Research*, Volume 48, No. 9, pp. 1933-1939 (1979).

John Curnette, et al., "Fluoride-mediated Activation of the Respiratory Burst in Human Neutrophils", *Journal of Clinical Investigation*, Volume 63, pp. 637-647 (1979).

W. L. Gabler, et al., "Effect of Fluoride on the Kinetics of Superoxide Generation by Fluoride", *Journal of Dental Research*, Volume 64, p. 281 (1985).

W. L. Gabler, et al., "Modulation of the Kinetics of Induced Neutrophil Superoxide Generation", *Journal of Dental Research*, Volume 65, pp. 1159-1165 (1986).

Takuya Saito, et al., "Effect of Heavy Metals on Functions of Mouse Phagocytic Cells", *Kankyo Kagaku Kenkyusho Kenku Hokuku (Kinki Daigaku)*, Volume 13, pp. 207-209 (1985).

A. S. Kozlyuk, et al., "Immune Status of Children in Chemically Contaminated Environments", *Zdravookhranenie*, Issue 3, pp. 6-9 (1987).

Alfred Taylor and Nell Carmichael Taylor, "Effect of Sodium Fluoride on Tumor Growth", *Proceedings of the Society for Experimental Biology and Medicine*, Volume 119, pp. 252-255 (1965).

[The following preliminary study indicates that fluoride inhibits antibody formation.]

S. K. Jain; A. K. Susheela, "Effect of sodium fluoride on antibody formation in rabbits", *Environmental Research*, Volume 44, pp. 117-125 (1987).

[The following preliminary study indicates that fluoride disrupts the adhesiveness of polymorphonucleocytes.]

J. L. Gomez-Ubric, et. al., "In vitro immune modulation of polymorphonuclear leukocyte adhesiveness by sodium fluoride", *Eur. J. Clin. Invest.*, Volume 22, pp. 659-661 (1992).

Chapter 4 Breaking Down the Body's Glue

L. Golub, et al., "The Effect of Sodium Fluoride on the Rates of Synthesis and Degradation of Bone Collagen in Tissue Culture", *Proceedings of the Society for Experimental Biology and Medicine*, Volume 129, pp. 973-977 (1968).

W. A. Peck, et al., "Fluoride Inhibition of Bone Collagen Synthesis", *Clinical Research*, Volume 13, pp. 330 (1965).

Kakuya Ishida, "The Effects of Fluoride on Bone Metabolism", *Koku Eisei Gakkai Zasshi*, Volume 31, No. 2, pp. 74-78 (1981).

Marian Drozdz, et al., "Studies on the Influence of Fluoride Compounds upon Connective Tissue Metabolism in Growing Rats", *Toxilogical European Research*, Volume 3, No. 5, pp. 237, 239-241 (1981).

Marian Drozdz, et al., "Studies on the Influence of Fluoride Compounds upon Connective Tissue Metabolism in Growing Rats. II Effect of Sodium Fluoride With and Without Simultaneous Exposure to Hydrogen Fluoride on Collagen Metabolism", *J. Toxicol. Med.*, Volume 4, pp. 151-157 (1984).

Anna Put, et al., "Effect of Chronic Administration of Sodium Fluoride and Calcium Carbonate on Some Biochemical Changes in Rats", *Bromatol. Chem. Toksykol.*, Volume 16, pp. 219-224 (1983).

Weislawa Jrzynka and Anna Put, "Effect of Chronic Fluoride Poisoning on the Morphological Appearance of Dentin in White Rats", *Czas. Stoma.*, Volume 37, pp. 169-175 (1984).

A.K. Susheela and Mohan Jha, "Effect of Fluoride on Cortical and Cancellous Bone Composition", *IRCS Medical Sciences: Library Compendium*, Volume 9, No. 11, pp. 1021-1022 (1981).

Y.D. Sharma, "Effect of Sodium Fluoride on Collagen Cross-link Precursors", *Toxicological Letters*, Volume 10, pp. 97-100 (1982).

A. K. Susheela and D. Mukerjee, "Fluoride poisoning and the Effect of Collagen Biosynthesis of Osseous and Nonosseous Tissue of Rabbit", *Toxicological European Research*, Volume 3, No. 2, pp. 99-104 (1981).

Y. D. Sharma, "Variations in the Metabolism and Maturation of Collagen after Fluoride Ingestion", *Biochimica et Biophysica Acta*, Volume 715, pp. 137-141 (1982).

Harold Fleming and Val Greenfield, "Changes in the Teeth and Jaws of Neonatal Webster Mice After Administration of Sodium Fluoride and Calcium Fluoride to the Female Parent During gestation", *Journal of Dental Research*, Volume 33, No. 6, pp. 780-788 (1954).

S. Chen and D. Eisenmann, "Calcium Shifts in Ameloblasts During Experimentally Altered Enamel Formation", *Journal of Dental Research*, Volume 6, p. 372 (1985).

John R. Farley, et al., "Fluoride Directly Stimulates Proliferation and Alkaline Phosphatase Activity of Bone Forming Cells," *Science*, Volume 222, pp. 330-332 (1983).

J.R. Smid, et al., "Effect of Long-Term Administration of Fluoride on the Levels of EDTA-Soluble Protein and Gamma Carboxyglutamic Acid in Rat Incisor Teeth", *Journal of Dental Research*, Volume 63, pp. 1061-1063 (1984).

J. H. Bowes and M. M. Murray, "A Chemical Study of 'Mottled Teeth' from Maldon, Essex", *British Dental Journal*, Volume 60, pp. 556-562 (1936).

Kh. A. Abishev, et al., "Molecular Composition of Bones During Chronic Fluoride Poisoning", *Zdravookr. Kaz*, Volume 30, No. 5, pp. 28-30 (1971).

B. R. Bhussry, "Chemical and Physical Studies of Enamel from Human Teeth", *Journal of Dental Research*, Volume 38, pp. 369-373 (1959).

S. Dajean; J. Menanteau, "A western-blotting study of enamel glycoproteins in rat experimental fluorosis", *Archives of Oral Biology*, Volume 34, pp. 413-418 (1989).

C. H. Weischer, et. al., "Effects of mellitic acid (MA) and sodium fluoride (NaF) on the histological appearance of murine fetal tibiae cultured in vitro", *Histol Histopathol*, Volume 1, pp. 303-308 (1986).

P. Chavassieux, et. al., "Dose effects on ewe bone remodeling of short-term sodium fluoride administration—a histomorphometric and biochemical study", *Bone*, Volume 12, pp. 421-427 (1991).

P. Chavassieux, et al., "Fluoride-induced bone changes in lambs during and after exposure to sodium fluoride", *Osteoporos. Int.*, Volume 2, pp. 26-31 (1991).

P. K. DenBesten and H. Thariani, "Biological mechanisms of fluorosis and level and timing of systemic exposure to fluoride with respect to fluorosis", *Journal of Dental Research,* Volume 71, pp. 1238-1243 (1992).

G.L. Chen, "Experimental study of antagonizing effect of calcium and magnesium against fluoride toxicity in collagen", *Chung Hua Yu Fang I Hsueh Tsa Chih*, Volume 26, pp. 80-82 (1992).

T. Sawadaet al., "Demonstration of amelogenins in globular bodies induced in rat-incisor secretory ameloblasts after fluoride administration", *Shika Kiso Igakkai Zasshi*, Volume 32, pp. 87-89 (1990).

N. Wakamatsu et al., "The crystallinity of hypomineralized rat enamel caused by fluoride administration", *Shoni Shikagaku Zasshi,* Volume 28, pp. 449-458 (1990).

JE. Harrison et al., "The effects of fluoride on ectopic bone formation", *J Bone Miner Res.,* Volume 5 (Suppl 1), pp 81-85 (1990).

S. Araki, "Ultrastructural changes in rat-incisor odontoblasts and dentin caused by administration of sodium fluoride", *Shikwa-Gakuho*, Volume 89, pp. 49-91 (1989).

M. Soriano, "Periostitis Deformans Due to Wine Fluorosis", *Fluoride,* Volume 1, pp. 56-64 (1968).

Chapter 5 The First Visible Sign of Fluoride Poisoning

A. Bronckers, et al., "A Histological Study of the Short-Term Effects of Fluoride on Enamel and Dentine Formation in Hamster Tooth-Germs in Organ Culture in Vitro", *Archives of Oral Biology,* Volume 29, pp. 803-810 (1984).

P.K. DenBesten and M.A. Crenshaw, "The Effects of Chronic High Fluoride Levels on Forming Enamel in Rats", *Archives of Oral Biology,* Volume 29, pp. 675-679 (1984).

P.K. DenBesten and H. Thariani, "Biological mechanisms of fluorosis and level and timing of systemic exposure to fluoride with respect to fluorosis", *Journal of Dental Research,* Volume 71, pp. 1238-1243 (1992).

A. Richards, et al., "Dental Fluorosis Developed During Stage of Enamel Maturation", *Journal of Dental Research,* Volume 64, p. 301 (1985).

Lanxing Li, et al., "Determination of Fluoride, Phosphorus and Calcium in Teeth after Fluoridation of Water Supply," *Zhonghua Kouqiangke Zazhi,* Volume 18, pp. 182-184 (1983).

S. Dajean and J. Menanteau, "A western-blotting study of enamel glycoproteins in rat experimental fluorosis", *Archives of Oral Biology,* Volume 34, pp. 413-418 (1989).

T. Sawada et al., "Demonstration of amelogenins in globular bodies induced in rat-incisor secretory ameloblasts after fluoride administration", *Shika. Kiso. Igakkai. Zasshi,* Volume 32, pp. 87-89 (1990).

N. Wakamatsu et al., "The crystallinity of hypomineralized rat enamel caused by fluoride administration", *Shika. Kiso. Igakkai. Zasshi,* Volume 28, pp 449-458 (1990).

Weislawa Jrzynka and Anna Put, "Effect of Chronic Fluoride Poisoning on the Morphological Appearance of Dentin in White Rats", *Czas. Stoma.,* Volume 37, pp. 169-175 (1984).

S. Araki, "Ultrastructural Changes in Rat-incisor Odontoblasts and Dentin Caused by Administration of Sodium Fluoride", *Shikwa. Gakuh,* Volume 89, pp. 49-91 (1989).

G.V. Black and Frederick McKay, "Mottled Teeth: An Endemic Developmental Imperfection of the Enamel of the Teeth, Heretofore Unknown in the Literature of Dentistry", *Dental Cosmos,* Volume 58, pp. 129-156 (1916).

Frederick McKay and G.V. Black, "An Investigation of Mottled Teeth: An Endemic Developmental Imperfection of the Enamel of Teeth, Hitherto Unknown in the Literature of Dentistry", *Dental Cosmos,* Volume 58, pp. 447-484 (1916).

Frederick McKay and G.V. Black, "An Investigation of Mottled Teeth: An Endemic Developmental Imperfection of the Enamel of Teeth, Heretofore Unknown in the Literature of Dentistry", *Dental Cosmos,* Volume 58, pp. 627-644 (1916).

Frederick McKay and G.V. Black, "An Investigation of Mottled Teeth: An Endemic Developmental Imperfection of the Enamel of the Teeth, Heretofore Unknown in the Literature of Dentistry", *Dental Cosmos,* Volume 58, pp. 781-792 (1916).

Frederick McKay and G.V. Black, "An Investigation of Mottled Teeth: An Endemic Developmental Imperfection of the Enamel of the Teeth, Heretofore Unknown in the Literature of Dentistry", *Dental Cosmos,* Volume 58, No. 2, pp. 894-904 (1916).

H.V. Churchill, "The Occurrence of Fluorides in Some Waters of the United States", *Journal of the American Water Works Association,* Volume 23, pp. 1399-1403 (1931).

M.C. Smith, et al., "The Cause of Mottled Enamel, a Defect of Human Teeth", *Technical Bulletin No. 32*, University of Arizona College of Agriculture, Tucson, Arizona, June 10, 1931.

H. Velu, "Dental Dystrophy in Mammals of the Phosphate Zone and Chronic Fluorosis", *C.R. Seances Soc. Biol. Ses. Fil.,* Volume 108, pp. 7450-752 (1931).

B.G. Anderson, "An Endemic Center of Mottled Enamel in China", *Journal of Dental Research,* Volume 12, pp. 591-593 (1932).

J. Chaneles, "A Dental Problem of Interest in Argentina: The Etiology of 'Mottled Teeth'", *Rev. Odontol. (Buenos Aires),* Volume 20, pp. 64-73 (1932).

N.J. Ainsworth, "Mottled Teeth", *British Dental Journal,* Volume 55, pp. 233-250 (1933).

E. Ricci, "The Phenomenon of Mottled Teeth in Italy", *Ann. Clinc. Odontol,* Volume 12, pp. 1029-1043 (1933).

R. Nakano, "A Statistical Observation of Endemic Effects on Teeth", *Rinsho Shika,* Volume 2, p. 102 (1933).

H. Trendley Dean and E. Elvove, "Further Studies on Minimal Threshold of Chronic Endemic Dental Fluorosis", *Public Health Reports,* Volume 52, pp. 1249-1264 (1937).

Vincent A. Segretto, et al., "A current Study of Mottled Enamel in Texas", *Journal of the American Dental Association,* Volume 108, pp, 56-59 (1984).

Dennis Leverett, "Fluorides and the Changing Prevalence of Decay Rates", *Science,* Volume 217, pp. 26-30 (1982).

Dennis Leverett, "Prevalence of Dental Fluorosis in Fluoridated and Nonfluoridated Communities", *Journal of Public Health Dentistry,* Volume 46, pp. 184-187 (1986).

John Colquhoun, "Disfiguring Dental Fluorosis in Auckland, New Zealand", *Fluoride,* Volume 17, pp. 234 (1984).

John Colquhoun, "Fluoridation in New Zealand, New Evidence Part 2", *American Laboratory,* Volume 17, pp. 98-109 (1985)

J.P. Brown, "Fluoride Supplements and Fluorosis of Enamel", *Journal of Dental Research,* Volume 64, p. 225 (1985).

R. Peters and A.G. Dreyer, "Safety considerations in topical fluoride therapy", *Tydskr. Tandheelkd. Ver. S. Afr.* Volume 46, pp. 183-186 (1991).

P.F. DePaola, "History of Fluoride Ingestion among Children Diagnosed with and without Fluorosis", *Journal of Dental Research,* Volume 64, p. 226 (1985).

M.J. Larsen, et al., "Development of Dental Fluorosis according to Age at Start of Fluoride Administration", *Caries Research,* Volume 19, pp. 519-527 (1985).

Maury Massler and Isaac Schour, "Relation of Endemic Dental Fluorosis to Malnutrition", *Journal of the American Dental Association,* Volume 44, pp. 156-165 (1952).

P.K. Debsten and M.A. Crenshaw, "Effects of Fluoride on Ameloblast Modulation", *Journal of Dental Research,* Volume 64, p. 373 (1984).

A. Richards, et al., "Dental Fluorosis Developed During State of Enamel Maturation", *Journal of Dental Research,* Volume 64, p. 301 (1985).

O. Fejerskov, et al., "Microradiography of the Effect of Acute and Chronic Administration of Fluoride on Human and Rat Dentine and Enamel", *Archives of Oral Biology,* Volume 24, pp. 123-130 (1979).

D.A. Timko, et al., "Effect of Fluoride on Calcium Uptake in Developing Enamel", *Journal of Dental Research,* Volume 64, p. 373 (1985).

R.S. Nanda, et al., "Factors Affecting the Prevalence of Dental Fluorosis in Lucknow, India", *Archives of Oral Biology,* Volume 19, pp. 781-792 (1974).

John Murray, "Adult Dental Health in Fluoride and Non-fluoride Areas", *British Dental Journal,* Volume 131, pp. 437-442 (1971).

Eugene Zimmerman, et al., "Oral Aspects of Excessive Fluorides in a Water Supply", *Journal of the American Dental Association,* Volume 50, pp. 272-277 (1955).

Chapter 6 Aging the Bone: The Degenerative Effects of Fluoride

T. R. Weingrad, "Periostitis due to low-dose fluoride intoxication demonstrated by bone scanning", *Clinic Nuclear Medicine,* Volume 16, pp 59-61 (1991).

Amarjit Singh and S.S. Jolly, "Chronic Toxic Effects on the Skeletal System", *Fluorides and Human Health,* World Health Organization, Geneva, Switzerland, 1970, pp. 238-249.

Amarjit Singh, et al., "Skeletal Changes in Endemic Fluorosis", *Journal of Bone and Joint Surgery,* Volume 44 B, No. 4, pp. 806-815 (1962).

V. N. Medvedeva, "The diagnosis and treatment of osteoarthrosis deformans in subjects in contact with fluorine compounds", *Vrach. Delo.* Volume 8, pp. 76-78 (1992).

S.S. Jolly, et al., "Endemic Fluorosis in Punjab", *Fluoride,* Volume 6, pp. 4-18 (1973).

M. R. C. Naidu, et al., "Skeletal Fluorosis Secondary to Occult Renal Disease", *Fluoride* 19: 166-168 (1986).

G. Boivin, et al., "Skeletal Fluorosis: Histomorphometric Analysis of Bone Changes and Bone Fluoride Content in 29 Patients", *Bone* Volume 10, pp. 89-99 (1989).

Arnold J. Felsenfeld and Mark E. Roberts, "A Report of Fluorosis in the United States Secondary to Drinking Well Water", *Journal of the American Medical Association* Volume 265, pp. 486-488 (1991)

J. C. Maloo, et al., "Fluorotic Radiculomyelopathy in a Libyan Male", *Clinical Neurology and Neurosurgery* , Volume 92, pp. 63-65 (1990).

H. Kudo, " Clinical and epidemiological study on osteofluorosis". *Nippon Eiseigaku Zasshi.* Volume 46, pp. 984-993 (1991).

G.N. Opinya and B. Imalingat, "Skeletal and dental fluorosis: two case reports", *East Afr Med J.* Volume 68, pp. 304-311 (1991).

B.S. Rao, "Ossification of the posterior longitudinal ligament and fluorosis", published erratum appears in *J Bone Joint Surg*, Volume 74, pp. 469-70, 629 (1992).

George Waldbott, et al., *Fluoridation: The Great Dilemma*, Coronado Press, Lawrence, Kansas, 1978, 423 pp.

J.A. Albright, "The Effect of Fluoride on the Mechanical Properties of Bone", *Transactions of the Annual Meeting of the Orthopedics Research Society,* pp. 3, 98 (1978).

B. Uslu, "Effect of Fluoride on Collagen Synthesis in the Rat", *Research in Experimental Medicine,* Volume 182, pp. 7-12 (1983).

Steven Jacobsen, et al., "Regional Variation in the Incidence of Hip Fracture", *Journal of the American Medical Association,* Volume 264, pp. 500-502 (1990).

Cyrus Cooper, et al., "Water Fluoridation and Hip Fracture", *Journal of the American Medical Association,* Volume 266, pp. 513-514 (1991) [this paper corrects inadequacies in a previous paper by Cooper published earlier in the *Journal of Epidemiology and Community Health*, Volume 44, pp. 17-19 (1990)].

C. Danielson et al., "Hip fractures and fluoridation in Utah's elderly population", *Journal of the American Medical Association.* Volume 268, pp. 746-748 (1992).

M.F. Sowers et al., "A prospective study of bone mineral content and fracture in communities with differential fluoride exposure", *Am. J. Epidemiol.*, Volume 133, pp. 649-660 (1991).

Lian Zong-Chen and Wu En-Huei, "Osteoporosis — An Early Radiographic Sign of Endemic Fluorosis", *Skeletal Radiology* , Volume 15, pp. 350-353 (1986).

Stephen Marks, "Restraint and Use of High-Dose Fluorides to Treat Skeletal Disorders," *Journal of the American Medical Association,* Volume 240, No. 15, pp. 1630-1631 (1978).

J.C. Robin, et al., "Studies on Osteoporosis III. Effect of Estrogens and Fluoride," *Journal of Medicine*, Volume 11, pp. 1-14 (1980).

J.C. Robin and J.L. Ambrus, "Studies on Osteoporosis IX. Effect of Fluoride on Steroid Induced Osteoporosis," *Research Communications in Chemical Pathology and Pharmacology*, Volume 37, No. 3, pp. 453-461 (1982).

C. M. Schnitzler, et al., "Histomorphometric Analysis of a Calcaneal Stress Fracture: A Possible Complication of Fluoride Therapy for Osteoporosis", *Bone*, Volume 7, pp. 193-198 (1986).

M. A. Dumbacher, et al., "Long-term Fluoride Therapy of Postmenopausal Osteoporosis", *Bone*, Volume 7, pp. 199-205 (1986).

B. Lawrence Riggs, "Effect of Fluoride Treatment on the Fracture Rate in Postmenopausal Women with Osteoporosis", *New England Journal of Medicine*, Volume 322, pp. 802-809 (1990).

C. M. Schnitzler et al., "Bone fragility of the peripheral skeleton during fluoride therapy for osteoporosis", *Clin. Orthop.*, Volume 261, pp. 268-275 (1990)

L. R. Hedlund and J. C. Gallagher, "Increased Hip Fractures in Osteoporotic Women Treated with Sodium Fluoride", *Journal of Bone and Mineral Research*, Volume 4, pp. 223-225 (1989).

C. Marcelli, et al., "Bone Complications during the Treatment of Osteoporosis with Fluoride", *Rev. Med. Interne*, Volume 10, pages 118-126 (1989).

V. Laurent, et al., "Bone Fluoride Determination in Osteoporotic Patients Treated with Sodium Fluoride", *Presse Med.*, Volume 18, pp. 679-682 (1989).

R. Duriez, et al., "Microradiographic Study of Iliac Bone Biopsies Taken after Treatment of Postmenopausal Osteoporosis with Sodium Fluoride", *Rev. Rheum. Mal. Osteoartic.*, Volume 56, pp. 375-381 (1989).

G. Weryha, et al "Bone complications of fluorotherapy: influence of androgen deficiency", *Ann Endocrinol Paris.* Volume 51, pp. 218-221 (1990).

P.B. Duell and C.H. Chesnut, "Exacerbation of rheumatoid arthritis by sodium fluoride treatment of osteoporosis", *Annals of Internal Medicine*, Volume 151, pp. 783-784 (1991).

Tina Weingrad, et al., "Periostitis due to Low-Dose Fluoride Intoxication Demonstrated by Bone Scanning", *Clin. Nucl. Med.*, Volume 16, pp. 59-61 (1991).

[According to the April 23, 1980 issue of the *Medical Tribune*, page 7, it was found that even low doses of fluoride in osteoporosis treatment cause rheumatic and gastrointestinal adverse reactions. Severe vomiting occurred in two patients until fluoride levels were reduced to 3.7 to 7.5 mg per day].

Paul Duffey, et al., "Giant Cells in Bone Marrows of Patients on High-Dose Fluoride Treatment", *Annals of Internal Medicine*, Volume 75, pp. 745-747 (1971).

P.E. Cordy, et al., "Bone Disease in Hemodialysis Patients with Particular Reference to the Effect of Fluoride in Study of Nutritional Requirements of Patients on Chronic Hemodialysis", *National Institute of Arthritis and Metabolic Diseases*, July 1973, pp. 218-59. [Distributed by the National Technical Information Service of the U.S. Department of Commerce].

L.J. Ream and P.B. Pendergrass, "The Effects of Fluoride on the Periosteal and Endosteal Surfaces of the Rat Femur", *Journal of Submicrosc. Cytology,* Volume 14, No. 1, pp. 81-91 (1982).

M. Soriano, "Periostitis Deformans Due to Wine Fluorosis", *Fluoride*, Volume 1, pp. 56-64 (1968).

A.F. Aksyuk and G.V. Bulychev, "Physiological Effects of Small Amounts of Fluoride on the Organism", *Gigiena i Sanitariya,* Volume 27, No. 12, pp. 7-10 (1962).

D.H. Retief, et al., "Fluoride Distribution in Enamel and Cementum of Human Fluorosed and Non-fluorosed Mandibular Molar Teeth", *Tandheelkd. Ver. s. Afr.,* Volume 39, pp. 243-246 (1984).

Chapter 7 Premature Aging: Skin, Arteries, Other Tissues

Amarjit Singh and S.S. Jolly, "Chronic Toxic Effects on the Skeletal System", in *Fluorides and Human Health*, World Health Organization, Geneva, Switzerland, 1970, pp. 238-249.

F. Pinet, et al., "Endemic Fluoride Bone Disorders from Drinking water - 49 Observations in South Algeria", *Annals of Radiology*, Volume 4, pp. 589-612 (1961).

S.P. Kumar and R.A.K. Harper, "Fluorosis in Aden", *British Journal of Radiology*, Volume 36, pp. 497-502 (1963).

M. Soriano, "Periostitis Deformans Due to Wine Fluorosis", *Fluoride*, Volume 1, pp. 56-64 (1968).

S. Chawla, et al., "Changes in Endemic Fluorosis", *Journal of the Association of Physicians - India*, Volume 80, pp. 429-433 (1945).

L. Seppa, et al., "Fluoride and Magnesium Intake in Relation to Atherosclerosis, Dental Caries and Rental Calculus in Rats", *Fluoride Metab., Proc. Satell. Symp. Int. Congr. Physiol. Sci.*, Volume 28, pp. 91-117 (1981).

J. Balic and A. Kansky "Skin telangiectasia in workers of an aluminium processing plant", *Derm. Beruf. Umwelt.,* Volume 20, pp. 20-22 (1988).

H. Mohr and J. Kragstrup "A histomorphometric analysis of the effects of fluoride on experimental ectopic bone formation in the rat", *Journal of Dental Research* Volume 70, pp. 957-960 (1991).

George Waldbott, et al., *Fluoridation: the Great Dilemma*, Coronado Press, Lawrence, Kansas, 1978, pp. 110-119, 135, 139, 144, 161.

A.K. Susheela and P. Kharb, "Aortic calcification in chronic fluoride poisoning: biochemical and electron microscopic evidence", *Exp. Mol. Pathol.*, Volume 53, pp. 72-80 (1990).

Chapter 8 Genetic Damage and Cancer

John Little, "Relationship Between DNA Repair Capacity and Cellular Aging", *Gerontology*, Volume 22, pp. 28-55 (1976).

Wolfgang Klein, et al., "DNA Repair and Environmental Substances", *Zeitschrift fur Angewandte Bader und Kilmaheilkunde*, Volume 24, No. 3, pp. 218-223 (1977).

Wolfgang Klein, et al., "Biochemical Research on the Action of Sodium Fluoride on Mammalian Cells. The Effect on Biosynthesis of Nucleic Acid and Proteins on Mouse Spleen Cells in in Vivo Studies", *Report of the Austrian Society of Atomic Energy, Seibersdorf Research Center*, No. 2355, pp. 1-10 (1974).

Wolfgang Klein, et al., "DNA Repair and Environmental Substances", *Report of the Austrian Society of Atomic Energy, Seibersdorf Research Center*, No. 2613, pp. 1-9 (1976).

S. I. Voroshilin, et al., "Cytogenetic Effect of Inorganic Fluorine Compounds on Human and Animal Cells in Vivo and in Vitro", *Genetika*, Volume 9, No. 4, pp. 115-120 (1973).

Georgianna Jagiello and Ja-Shein Lin, "Sodium Fluoride as Potential Mutagen in Mammalian Eggs", *Archives of Environmental Health*, Volume 29, pp. 230-235 (1974).

Danuta Jachimczak and Bogumila Skotarczak, "The Effect of Fluorine and Lead Ions on the Chromosomes of Human Leucocytes in Vitro", *Genetica Polonica*, Volume 19, No. 3, pp. 353-357 (1978).

George Martin, et al., "Lack of Cytogenetic Effect in Mice or Mutations in Salmonella Receiving Sodium Fluoride", *Mutation Research*, Volume 66, pp. 159-167 (1979).

A. A. Aliev and D. A. Babaev, "Cytogenetic Activity of Vitamins in Bone Marrow Cells of Rat Femurs in Sodium Fluoride-Induced Mutation Conditions", *Tsitol. Genet.*, Volume 15, pp. 19-23 (1981).

A. A. Aliev, et al., "Effect of alpha-Tocopherol on the Level of Chromosome Aberrations Induced by Sodium Fluoride in Rat Femur Bone Marrow Cells", *Izv. Akad. Nauk Az. SSR Serv. Biol. Naul.*, No. 1, pp. 17-20 (1981).

V Yu Akhundov, et al., "Effect of Combined and Separate Exogenous Vitamin Administration of the Level of Chromosomal Aberrations Induced by Sodium Fluoride in Rats in Subacute Experiments", *Izv. Akad. Nauk Az. SSR, Ser. Biol. Nauk*, No. 4, pp. 3-5 (1981).

Aly Mohamed and M. E. Chandler, "Cytological Effects of Sodium Fluoride on Mice", *Fluoride*, Volume 15, No. 3, pp. 110-118 (1983).

W. He et al., "Effect of fluoride and fluoroacetamide on sister chromatid exchanges and chromosomal aberrations in cultured red Muntjac (Muntjacus muntjac) cells", *Huangjing Kexue Xuebao*, Volume 3, pp. 94-100 (1983).

Takeki Tsutsui, et al., "Sodium Fluoride-induced Morphological and Neoplastic Transformation, Chromosome Aberrations, Sister Chromatid Exchanges, and Unscheduled DNA Synthesis in Cultured Syrian Hamster Embryo Cells", *Cancer Research*, Volume 44, pp. 938-941 (1984).

Takeki Tsutsui, et al., "Cytotoxicity, Chromosome Aberrations and Unscheduled DNA Synthesis in Cultured Human Diploid Fibroblasts Induced by Sodium Fluoride", *Mutation Research*, Volume 139, pp. 193-198 (1984).

K. Kishi and A. Tonomura, "Mutagenicity of sodium fluoride - review and human lymphocyte assay", *Husso Kenkyu* , Volume 5, pp. 35-41 (1984).

E. J. Thompson, et al., "The Effect of Fluoride on Chromosome Aberration and Sister-Chromatid Exchange Frequencies in Cultured Human Lymphocytes", *Mutation Research*, Volume 144, pp. 89-92.

J. Cole et al. "The mutagenicity of sodium fluoride to L5178Y [wild type and TK +/- (3.7.2c)] mouse lymphoma cells", *Mutagenesis,* Volume 1, pp. 157-167 (1986).

D. Scott and S. A. Roberts, "Extrapolation from in vitro tests to human risks: experience with sodium fluoride clastogenicity", *Mutation Research*, Volume 189, pp. 47-58 (1987).

W. J. Caspary et al., "Mutagenic activity of fluorides in mouse lymphoma cells", *Mutation Research*, Volume 187, pp. 165-180 (1987).

R. Albanese, "Sodium fluoride and chromosome damage (in vitro human lymphocyte and in vivo micronucleus analysis)", *Mutagenesis*, Volume 2, pp. 497-499 (1987).

S. Tazhibaev et al., "A Modifying effect of nutrition on the mutagenic activity of phosphorus and fluorine compounds", *Vopr Pritan* , Volume 4, pp. 63-66 (1987).

M.J. Aardema et al. "Sodium fluoride-induced chromosomes aberrations in different stages of the cell cycle: a proposed mechanism", *Mutation Research*, Volume 223, pp. 191-203 (1989).

N. Suzuki and T. Tsutsui, "Dependence of lethality and incidence of chromosome aberrations induced by treatment of synchronized human diploid fibroblasts with sodium fluoride on different periods of the cell cycle", *Shigaku*, Volume 77, pp. 436-447 (1989).

A.H. Mohammed, et al., "Cytological Reactions Induced by Sodium Fluoride in Allium Cepa Root-Tip Chromosomes", *Canadian Journal of Genetics and Cytology*, Volume 8, pp. 241-244 (1966).

A.H. Mohamed, et al., "Cytological Effects on Hydrogen Fluoride on Tomato Chromosomes", *Canadian Journal of Genetics and Cytology*, Volume 8, pp. 575-583 (1966).

A. H. Mohamed, "Cytogenetic Effects of Hydrogen Fluoride Treatment in Tomato Plants", *Journal of the Air Pollution Control Association*, Volume 18, pp. 395-398 (1968).

A.H. Mohamed, "Chromosome Changes in Maize Induced by Fluoride Gas", *Canadian Journal of Genetics and Cytology*, Volume 12, pp. 614-620 (1970).

A.H. Mohamed, "Induced Recessive Lethals in Second Chromosomes in Drosophila Melanogaster by Hydrogen Fluoride", *Proceedings of the Second International Clear Air Congress of the International Union of Air Pollution Prevention Associations*, 1970, p. 26.

R.A. Gerdes, et al., "The Effects of Atmospheric Hydrogen Fluoride upon Drosophila Melanogaster", *Atmospheric Environ.*, Volume 5, pp. 113-122 (1971).

B. Mitchell and R.A. Gerdes, "Mutagenic Effects of Sodium Fluoride and Stannous Fluoride on Drosophila Melanogaster", *Fluoride*, Volume 6, pp. 113-117 (1973).

E. Vogel, "Strong Antimutagenic Effects of Fluoride on Mutation Induction by Trenimon and 1-Phenyl-3, 3-Dimethyltraizene in Drosophila Melanogaster", *Mutation Research*, Volume 20, pp. 339-352 (1973).

S.S. Bale and G.E. Hart "Studies on the cytogenetic and genetic effects of fluoride on barley. I A comparative study of the effects of sodium fluoride and hydrofluoric acid on seedling root tips", *Canadian Journal of Genetics and Cytology* , Volume 15, pp. 695-702 (1973).

S.S. Bale and G.E. Hart, "Cytogenetic and Genetic Effects of Fluoride on Barley, II. Effects of Treatments of Seedlings Coleoptiles with Sodium Fluoride", *Canadian Journal of Genetics and Cytology*, Volume 15, pp. 703-712 (1973).

A.A. Aliev, et al., "Cytogenetic Effect of Sodium Fluoride Treatment of Allium Fistulosum L. Seeds", *Izv. Akad. Nauk Az. SSR,* Ser. Biol. Nauk, No. 2, pp. 8-10 (1982).

P. C. Pati et al., "Features of the Modifying Capacity of Mutations in Aegilops Seed Produced Under Various Ecological Conditions", *Izv. Akad. Nauk Az. SSR*, Ser. Biol. Nauk, No. 4, pp. 21-24 (1983).

R.N. Mukherjee and F.H. Sobels, "The Effect of Sodium Fluoride and Iodoacetamide on Mutation Induction by X-Irradiation in Mature Spermatozoa of Drosophila", *Mutation Research*, Volume 6, pp. 217-225 (1968).

A. Iarez, et al., "Sodium Fluoride, Fetotoxicity, and Oral Experimental Teratogeny in Rats", Toxicological Aspects in [9th Annual Symposium of the International Congress of the European Association of Poison Control Centers], 1981, pp. 528-540.

Ruitao Zhang and Shunguang Zhang, "Toxicity of Fluoride to Fish", *Huangjing Kexue*, Volume 3, pp. 1-5 (1983).

L. Du, "The effect of fluorine on the developing human brain", *Chung-hua-Ping-Li-Hsueh-Tsa-Chih*, Volume 21, pp. 218-220 (1992).

Stephen Greenberg, "The Reaction of Mouse Leukocytes to Long-Term Fluoride Exposure", *Anatomical Record*, Volume 196, No. 2, pp. 266-267 (1980).

Stephen Greenberg, "Leukocyte Response in Young Mice Chronically Exposed to Fluoride", *Fluoride*, Volume 15, No. 3, pp. 119-123 (1982).

[Listed below are some additional related references:

Nobutake Kanematsu, "Genetic Toxicity of Biomaterial. DNA Damaging Effects of Sodium Fluoride and Other Fluoride Compounds", *Japanese Journal of Oral Biology*, Volume 27, pp. 372-374 (1985).

V. Ya. Nikiforova, "Mechanism of the Mutagenic Action of Fluoride", *Tsitol. Genet.*, Volume 16, pp. 40-42 (1982).

Takeki Tsutsui, et al., "Induction of Unscheduled DNA Synthesis in Cultured Human Oral Keratinocytes by Sodium Fluoride", *Mutation Research*, Volume 140, pp. 43-48 (1984).

Qiyue Hu and Shoupeng Zhu, "Induction of Chromosomal Aberrations in Male Mouse Germ Cells by Uranyl Fluoride Containing Enriched Uranium", *Mutation Research*, Volume 224, pp. 209-214 (1990).

O. V. Zolotova and B. A. Petrov, "Assessment of total mutagenic activity of harmful factors of the industrial environment at the metallurgy plants of South Ural.", *Vestn. Ross. Akad. Med. Nauk.*, Volume 4, pp. 59-60, (1992).

L.S. Strochkova, et al., "Effect of Fluoride on Morphological and Metabolic Modifications in Hela Cell Culture", *Tsitologiya*, Volume 26, pp. 299-306 (1984).

Toshio Imai, et al., "Effects of Fluoride on Cell Growth of Two Human Cell Lines and on DNA and Protein Synthesis in Hela Cells", *Acta Pharmacol. Toxicol.*, Volume 52, pp. 8-11 (1983).

Kataoka Masayuki, "Effect of Sodium Fluoride on Blastogenesis in Mouse Lymphocytes with Special Reference to the Uptake on 3H-Thymidine, 3H-Uridine, or 3H-Leucine", *Shika Gakuho*, Volume 84, pp. 229-251 (1984).

Chong Chang, "Effect of Fluoride on Nucleotides and Ribonucleic Acid in Germinating Corn Seedling Roots", *Plant Physiology*, Volume 43, No. 5, pp. 669-674 (1968).

V.I. Shepotinovsky and Z.I. Mikashinovich, "Metabolic Response of Leukocytes as an Indicator of Animal Individual Reaction to Stress and Injury-Induced Shock", *Byull. Eksp. Biol. Med.*, Volume 90, No. 10, pp. 420-442 (1980).

Armando Moucdy, "Histochemical (Glycogen, RNA, and Lipids) Studies of the Liver Cells of Rats Treated with Potable Water Containing Sodium Fluoride in Various Concentrations", *Rev. Fac. Odontol, Univ. Sao Paulo*, Volume 5, No. 3, pp. 197-215 (1968).

George Waldbott, et al., "Genetic Damage, Birth Defects, and Cancer", *Fluoridation: the Great Dilemma*, Coronodo Press, pp. 209-238. (1978).]

Chapter 9 Cancer

Takeki Tsutsui, et al., "Sodium Fluoride-induced Morphological and Neoplastic Transformation, Chromosome Aberrations, Sister Chromatid Exchanges, and Unscheduled DNA Synthesis in Cultured Syrian Hamster Embryo Cells", *Cancer Research*, Volume 44, pp. 938-941 (1984).

C.A. Jones, et al., "Sodium fluoride promotes morphological transformation of Syrian hamster embryo cells", *Carcinogenesis*, Volume 9, pp. 2279-2284 (1988).

C. Lasne, et al. "Transforming activities of sodium fluoride in cultured Syrian hamster embryo and BALB/3T3 cells", *Cell Biol Toxicol*, Volume 4, pp. 311-324 (1988).

Irwin Herskowitz and Isabel Norton, "Increased Incidence of Melanotic Tumors in Two Strains of Drosophila Melanogaster Following Treatment with Sodium Fluoride", *Genetics*, Volume 48, pp. 307-310 (1963).

Paul Duffey, et al., "Giant Cells in Bone Marrows of Patients on High-Dose Fluoride Treatment", *Annals of Internal Medicine*, Volume 75, pp. 745-747 (1971).

A. Taylor and N.C. Taylor "Effect of fluoride on tumor growth", *Proceedings of the Society of Experimental Biology and Medicine* , Volume 65, pp. 252-255 (1965).

Dean Burk and J.A. Yiamouyiannis, "Fluoride and Cancer", *Congressional Record*, pp. H7173-H7176 (July 21, 1975).

J.A. Yiamouyiannis and Dean Burk, "Cancer From Our Drinking Water?" *Congressional Record*, pp. H12731-12734 (December 16, 1975).

J.A. Yiamouyiannis and Dean Burk, "Fluoridation of Public Water Systems and Cancer Death Rate in Humans", presented at the *67th Annual Meeting of Amer. Soc. biol. Chemists. Fed. Amer. Soc. Exp. Biol.* (June 1976).

J.A. Yiamouyiannis, "Fluoridation of Drinking Water and Cancer", *Lebensschultz*, Volume 3, No. 3, pp. 421-43 (1976).

J.A. Yiamouyiannis, "Relationship between Fluoridation of Drinking Water and Increase in Cancer Death Rate", *Der Naturartz*, Volume 98, No. 7, pp. 216-218 (1976).

J.A. Yiamouyiannis and Dean Burk, "Fluoridation and Cancer: Age Dependence of Cancer Mortality Related to Artificial Fluoridation", *Fluoride*, Volume 10, No. 3, pp. 102-123 (1977).

Letter from Donald Frederickson, Director of the National Institute of Health to Rep. Daniel Flood, December 4, 1975.

The National Cancer Program (Part 2. Fluoridation of Public Drinking Water), Hearing before a Subcommittee of the Committee on Government Operations, 95th Congress, 1st Session, September 21 and October 12, 1977, GPO 99-316-0, 580 pp. (1977).

J. David Erickson, *McColl vs. Strathclyde Regional Council*, Scottish High Court in Edinburgh, Exhibit 403 (1981).

Decision of *Paul W. Aitkenhead vs. Borough of West View* in the Court of Common Pleas of Allegheny County, Pennsylvania, No. DG4585-78 (1978).

Decision of *Illinois Pure Water vs. Director of the Department of Public Health of the State of Illinois*, in the Third Judicial Circuit, Madison County, No. 56315 (1982).

John Yiamouyiannis, "Fluoridation-linked Cancer Deaths Per 100,000 Population Corrected for Age, Race, and Sex", [Data refer to the difference in the observed cancer death rate and the expected cancer death rate of the fluoridated cities minus that of the nonfluoridated cities listed on the first page of Chapter 9. The standard population used is the U.S. population for 1950. All figures are based on normalization of the difference of 1940-1950 baseline figures to zero.]

Health Action, Volume 2, Nos. 11-12 (1981) 64 pp.

The National Cancer Program (Part 2. Fluoridation of Public Drinking Water), *Hearing before a Subcommittee of the Committee on Government Operations*, 95th Congress, 1st Session, September 21 and October 12, 1977, GPO 99-316-0, 580 pp. (1977).

The National Cancer Program (Part 2. Fluoridation of Public Drinking Water), *Hearing before a Subcommittee of the Committee on Government Operations*, 95th Congress, 1st Session, September 21 and October 12, 1977, GPO 99-316-0, p. 319.

J. Toft, *Sodium Fluoride: individual animal tumor pathology table [mice]*. Columbus, OH: Battelle Memorial Institute, 1989.

Persing R. Sodium, *Fluoride: individual animal tumor pathology table [rats]*. Columbus, OH: Battelle Memorial Institute, 1989.

R.N. Hoover et al, "Fluoridation of Drinking Water and Subsequent Cancer Incidence and Mortality", *Review of Fluoride: Benefits and Risks*, Report of the Ad Hoc Committee on Fluoride of the Committee to Coordinate Environmental Health and Related Programs, United States Public Health Service, DHHS, 1991 Feb: E1-E51.

Procter and Gamble. Carcinogenicity studies with sodium fluoride. Presented at the *National Institute of Environmental Health Sciences,* July 27, 1985

J. K. Maurer et al., "Two-year carcinogenicity study of sodium fluoride in rats", *J Nat Cancer Inst* ., Volume 82, pp. 1118-1126 (1990).

"Dose determination and carcinogenicity studies of sodium fluoride in Crl:CD-1 mice and Crl:CD (Sprague Dawley) BR rats" in *Review of Fluoride: Benefits and Risks*. Report of the Ad Hoc Committee on Fluoride of the Committee to Coordinate Environmental Health and Related Programs, United States Public Health Service, DHHS, 1991 Feb; 74 and D1-D7.

R.N. Hoover et al., "Time trends for bone and joint cancers and osteosarcomas in the Surveillance, Epidemiology and End Results (SEER) Program." In: *Review of Fluoride: Benefits and Risks*. Report of the Ad Hoc Committee on Fluoride of the Committee to Coordinate Environmental Health and Related Programs, United States Public Health Service, DHHS, 1991 Feb: F1-F7

P. D. Cohn, *A Brief Report on the Association of Drinking Water Fluoridation and the Incidence of Osteosarcoma among Young Males*, New Jersey Department of Health, Trenton, NJ, 1992 Nov

K.C. Kanwar, et al., "In vitro Inhibition of Testosterone Synthesis in the Presence of Fluoride Ions", *IRCS Med. Sci. Libr. Compend.*, Volume 11, pp. 813-814 (1983).

J. A. Yiamouyiannis, "Fluoridation and Cancer: The Biology and Epidemiology of Bone and Oral Cancer Related to Fluoridation", *Fluoride*, Volume 26, pages 83-96 (1993).

T. J. Mason and F.W. McKay, "Cancer Mortality by County: 1950 to 1969", publication no. (NIH) 74-615. *U.S. National Cancer Institute*, DHEW, 1974.

E. R. Schlesinger ER, et al. "Newburgh-Kingston caries-fluorine study. XIII. Pediatric findings after ten years", *J Amer Dent Assn* , Volume 52, pp. 296-306 (1956).

J. Caffey, "On fibrous defects in cortical walls: their radiologic appearance, structure, prevalence, natural course, and diagnostic significance", *In Advances in Pediatrics: Levin SZ,* pp. 13-51 (1955).

Drinking Water and Health. *National Academy of Sciences.* 1977, p. 388-389

N.N. Litvinov, et al., "Morbidity and Mortality in Man Caused by Pulmonary Cancer and Its Relation to the Pollution of the Atmosphere in the Areas of Aluminum Plants", *Acta Unionis Internationalis Contra Cancrum*, Volume 19, pp. 742-745 (1963).

V.A. Cecilioni, "Lung Cancer in a Steel City-Its Possible Relation to Fluoride Emissions", *Fluoride*, Volume 5, pp. 172-181 (1972).

P. Grandjean, et al., "Mortality and Cancer Morbidity after Heavy Occupational Fluoride Exposure", *American Journal of Edpdemiology*, Volume 121, pp. 57-67 (1985).

P. Grandjean et al., "Cancer incidence and mortality in workers exposed to fluoride", *J. Natl. Cancer. Inst.*, Volume 84, pp. 1903-1909 (1992).

T. Okamura and T. Matshuisa, "The Fluorine Content in Favorite Foods of Japanese", *Japan Journal of Public Health*, Volume 14, pp. 41-47 (1967).

Y. Z. Huang, et al, "Syndrome of endemic arsenism and fluorosis. A clinical study", *Chin. Med. J. Engl.*, Volume 105, pp. 586-590 (1992).

J. L. Shupe et al., "The pathology of chronic bone fluorosis: a review", *Toxicol Pathol.*, Volume 20, pp. 274-285 (1992).

Donald Austin, "Analyses Testing the Hypothesis that Fluoride in Drinking Water is Related to Cancer in Humans", *Hearings Before a Subcommittee of the Committee on Government Operations, House of Representatives*, 95th Congress, First Session, The National Cancer Program (Part 2, Fluoridation of Public Drinking Water), pp. 394-399 (1977).

Victor Cecilioni, " A Link Between Fluoridation and Excess Cancer Death Rates?" *Hearings Before a Subcommittee of the Committee on Government Operations, House of Representatives*, 95th Congress, First Session, The National Cancer Program (Part 2, Fluoridation of Public Drinking water), pp. 258-261 (1977).

J. David Erickson, "Mortality in Selected Cities with Fluoridated and Non-Fluoridated Water Supplies", *New England Journal of Medicine*, Volume 298, pp. 1112-1116 (1978).

John W. Knutson, "An Evaluation of the Grand Rapids Water Fluoridation Project", *Fluoride Drinking Waters*, pp. 213-217 (1962).

John Yiamouyiannis, "Fluoridation-linked Deaths Corrected for Age, Race, and Sex", [Data refer to the difference in the observed cancer death rate and the expected cancer death rate of the fluoridated cities minus that of the nonfluoridated cities listed on the first page of Chapter 9. The standard population used is the U.S. Population for 1950. The 3-4% increase in total mortality is based on a linear regression of figures from 1950 to 1968].

Chapter 10 The Prime Target

Fluorides, National Academy of Sciences, 1971, pp. 70-73.

Fluorides and Human Health, World Health Organization, Geneva, Switzerland, 1970, p. 183.

Alan Wiseman, "Effects of Inorganic Fluoride on Enzymes" in *Handbook of Experimental Pharmacology*, Volume 20, Part 2, Springer-Verlag, New York, pp. 48-97 (1970).

F. Maley and G.F. Maley, "The Presence of Deoxycytidylate Deaminase in Normal Adult Rat Liver", *Biochimica et Biophysica Acta*, Volume 47, pp. 181-183 (1961).

G. Cimasoni, "Further Observations Upon the Mechanism of Cholinesterase Inhibition by Fluoride Ion", *Journal of Dental Research*, Volume 44, P. 144 (1965).

E.A. Thibodeau, et al., "pH-Dependent Inhibition of Peroxidase Activity", *Journal of Dental Research*, Volume 64, pp. 1211-1213 (1985).

Reference Man, International Commission on Radiological Protection, Publication No. 23, Pergammon Press, New York, 1975, pp. 290-291, 300-301.

R.A. Call, et al., "Histological and Chemical Studies in Man on Effects of Fluoride", *Public Health Reports*, Volume 80, No. 6, pp. 529-538 (1965).

Alexander Gettler and Lester Ellerbrook, "Toxicology of Fluorides", *American Journal of Medical Science*, Volume 197, pp. 625-638 (1939).

F. Geeraerts, et al., unpublished data, 1986.

D.W.A. Roberts, "The Wheat Leaf Phosphates", *Canadian Journal of Biochemistry and Physiology*, Volume 41, pp. 113-120 (1963).

W.L. Traxel and V.S. LeQuire, "In Vitro Activation of Lipolytic Activity in the Serum of Dogs by Bile Salts", *Proceedings of the Society for Experimental Biology and Medicine*, Volume 116, pp. 388-392 (1964).

Chapter 11 How Fluoride Works

John Emsley, et al., " An Unexpectedly Strong Hydrogen Bond: Ab Initio Calculations and Spectroscopic Studies of Amide-Fluoride Systems", *Journal of the American Chemical Society*, Volume 103, pp. 24-28 (1981).

James H. Clark and Joseph Sherwood Taylor, "I.R. Evidence for a Strong Hydrogen Bond in the Fluoride-Uracil System", *Journal of the Chemical Society, Chemical Communications*, pp. 466-468 (1981).

Steven L. Edwards, et al., "The Crystal Structure of Fluoride-Inhibited Cytochrome c Peroxidase", *Journal of Biological Chemistry*, Volume 259, pp. 12984-1212988 (1984).

H.C. Froede and I. B. Wilson, "The Slow Rate of Inhibition of Acetylcholines-terase by Fluoride", *Molecular Pharmacology*, Volume 27, pp. 630-633 (1985).

1983 Physician's Desk Reference, Medical Economics Company, 1983, pp. 1976-1977.

1983 USPDI - Drug Information for the Health Care Provider, Volume I, United States Pharmacopeial Convention, 1982, pp. 805-807.

1983 USPDI - Advice for the Patient, Volume II, United States Pharmacopeial Convention, 1982, pp. 656-657.

John Emsley, et al., "The Uracil-Fluoride Interaction: Ab Initio Calculations Including Solvation", *Journal of the Chemical Society, Chemical Communications*, pp. 476-478 (May 1982).

"Hydrogen Bonds Show Their Strength", *New Scientist*, Volume 89, p. 211 (1981).

Chapter 12 How to Avoid Fluoride

O. Lantz, et al., "Fluoride-induced chronic renal failure", *Amer. J. Kidney Dis.*, Volume 10, pp. 136-9 (1987).

G. Boivin, et al., "Skeletal Fluorosis: Histomorphometric Analysis of Bone Changes and Bone Fluoride Content in 29 Patients", *Bone* , Volume 10, pp. 89-99 (1989).

J. G. Stannard et al., "Fluoride levels and fluoride contamination of fruit juices", *J. Clin. Pediatr. Dent.* Volume 16, pp. 38-40 (1991).

D. T. Pang et al., "Fluoride intake from beverage consumption in a sample of North Carolina children", *Journal of Dental Research* Volume 71, pp. 1382-1383 (1992).

Fluoride, Teeth & Health, A Report of the Royal College of Physicians, Pitman Medical, 1976, pp. 21-22.

S. Sergio Gomez, et al., "Fluoride content of tea and amount ingested by children", *Odontol. Chil.,* Volume 37, pp. 251-255 (1989).

C. Fraysse et al., "The role of tea consumption in dental fluorosis in Jordan", *Bull. Group. Int. Rech. Sci. Stomatol. Odontol.* Volume 32, pp. 39-46 (1989).

G. N. Opinya et al., "Fluorosis of deciduous teeth and first permanent molars in a rural Kenyan community", *Acta. Odontol. Scand.,* Volume 49, pp. 197-202 (1991).

J. H. Woltgens, et al., "Prevalence of Mottled Enamel in Permanent Dentition of Children Participating in a Fluoride Programme at the Amsterdam Dental School", *J. Biol. Buccale*, Volume 17, pp. 15-20 (1989).

M. W. Woolfolk, et al., "Relation of Sources of Systemic Fluoride to Prevalence of Dental Fluorosis", *Journal of Public Health Dentistry*, Volume 49, pp. 78-82 (1989).

R. S. Levin, et al., "A Photographically Recorded Assessment of Enamel Hypoplasia in Fluoridated and Non-Fluoridated Areas in England", *British Dental Journal*, Volume 166, pp. 249-252 (1989).

A.S. Lykova, et al., "Effect of Diets Containing Fluorine-Ion on Some Biochemical and Hematological Indicators of the Body", *Voprosy Pitaniia,* Volume 6, No. 6, pp. 46-47 (1981).

[The total fluoride intake has increased sharply over the last 30 years. The following is a list of studies which show that fluoride overdose among children and adults is now a concern; even the American Dental Association has been forced to admit that 1/2-mg fluoride supplements given to children by dentists and pediatricians are causing dental fluorosis. The Canadian Dental Association has gone even further and has advised that no fluoride supplements should be given to children under the age of three under any circumstances.]

Dyson Rose and John Marier, Environmental Fluoride 1977, *National Research Council of Canada*, Ottawa, Canada, 151 pp., (1977).

Elise Jerard and J.B. Patrick, "The Summing of Fluoride Exposures", *International Journal of Environmental Studies*, Volume 4, pp. 1441-155 (1973).

Robert Fand, "Medical Aspects of Fluoride and Fluorosis", *International Journal of Environmental Studies*, Volume 5, pp. 87-92 (1973).

John Lee, "Optimal Fluoridation", *Western Journal of Medicine*, Volume 122, pp. 431-436 (1975).

Dennis Leverett, "Fluorides and the Changing Prevalence of Dental Caries", *Science*, Volume 217, pp. 26-30 (1982).

R.H.S., "Editorial, Concern about Dietary Fluoride Supplementation", *Journal of American Dental Association*, Volume 96, p. 1158 (1978).

Yoshitsugu Imai, "Relation between Fluoride Concentration in Drinking Water and Dental Caries in Japan", *Koku Eisei Gakkai Zasshi*, Volume 22, No. 2, pp. 144-146 (1972).

T. Burkov and T. Burkova, "Early Morphological and Some Histochemical Enzyme Changes in the Liver and Oral Mucosa Produced by Fluoride-Containing Mineral Waters", *Nauchno-Izledovatelskiya Stomatologichen Institut*, Volume 13, pp. 1-9 (1969).

A.A. Petina and L.N. El'nichnykh, "Toxicological Characteristics of Fluorine during Its Simultaneous Entrance into an Organism Along With Drinking Water and Inhaled Air. II.", *Flyuoroz Ego Profl.*, Mater, Simp. 1966 (published 1967), pp. 157-163.

Chapter 13 The First Fable: Fluoride is Essential

"Is Fluorine an Essential Element?" *Fluorides*, National Academy of Sciences, Washington, D.C., pp. 66-68 (1971).

Richard Maurer and Harry Day, "The Non-Essentiality of Fluorine in Nutrition", *Journal of Nutrition*, Volume 62, pp. 561-573 (1957).

A.A. Doberenz, et al., "Minimal Fluoride Diet and Effect on Rats", *Federation Proceedings*, Volume 22, p. 554 (1963).

Klaus Schwarz and David Milne, "Fluorine Requirement for Growth in the Rat", *Bioinorganic Chemistry*, Volume 1, pp. 331-338 (1972).

Klaus Schwarz, "Recent Dietary Trace Element Research, Exemplified by Tin, Fluorine, and Silicon", *Federation Proceedings*, Volume 33, No. 6, pp. 1748-1757 (1974).

F.H. Nielsen and H.H. Sandstead, "Are Nickel, Vanadium, Silicon, Fluorine, and Tin Essential for Man", *American Journal of Clinical Nutrition*, Volume 27, pp. 515-520 (1974).

H.H. Messer, et al., "Influence of Fluoride Intake on Reproduction in Mice", *Journal of Nutrition*, Volume 103, pp. 1319-1326 (1973).

H.H. Messer and J.W. Suttie, "Discussion" in *Trace Element Metabolism in Animals-2*, University Park Press (Baltimore), 1974, pp. 435-437.

S. Tao and J.W. Suttie, "Evidence for a Lack of an Effect of Dietary Fluoride Level on Reproduction in Mice", *Journal of Nutrition*, Volume 106, pp. 115-1122 (1976).

S.W.J. van Rensburg and W.H. de Vos, "The Influence of Excess Fluorine Intake in Drinking Water on Reproductive Efficiency in Bovines", *Onderstepoort Journal of Veterinary Research*, Volume 33, No. 1, pp. 185-194 (1966).

K.C. Kanwar, et al., "In vitro Inhibition of Testosterone Synthesis in the Presence of Fluoride Ions", *IRCS Med. Sci. Libr. Compend.*, Volume 11, pp. 813-814 (1983).

F.I. Mandrik and Yu. L. Yakabouskaya, "Embroyotoxicity of Fluorine", *Veterinariya Moscow*, Number 11, pp. 66-67 (1984).

N. J. Chinoy, et al., "Microdose vasal injection of sodium fluoride in the rat", *Reprod-Toxicol.*, Volume 5, pp. 505-512 (1991).

N. J. Chinoy and E. Sequeira, "Effects of fluoride on the histoarchitecture of reproductive organs of the male mouse", *Reprod-Toxicol.*, Volume 3, pp. 261-267 (1989).

A. Krasowska and T. Wlostowski, "The effect of high fluoride intake on tissue trace elements and histology of testicular tubules in the rat", *Comp. Biochem. Physiol.-C*, Volume 103, pp. 31-34 (1992).

C.W. Weber and B.L. Reid, "Effect of Low-Fluoride Diets Fed to Mice for Six Generations", Trace Element Metabolism in Animals-2, *University Park Press (Baltimore)*, 1974, pp. 707-709.

A.I. Genkin, et al., "Effect of Chronic Fluoride Poisoning on Oxidative Processes in Body Tissues", *Farmakol. Tolsikol.* (Moscow), Volume 46, pp. 97-99 (1983).

T.D. Grekhova, "Effect of Hydrogen Fluoride on Adenine Nucleotide Contents in Blood Erythrocytes and Organs of White Rats", *Gig. Tr. Prof. Zabol.*, No. 5, pp. 43-44 (1984).

V.A. Shugaev, "Oxygen Balance and the Effect of Antihypoxic Drugs during Fluorine Intoxication", *Farmakol. Toksikol.* (Moscow), No. 47, pp. 94-97 (1984).

V.A. Shugaev, "Therapeutic and Prophylactic Effect of Glutamic Acid in Inhalation Poisoning with Fluoride Inorganic Compounds", *Gig. Tr. Prof. Zakol.*, No. 12, pp. 28-29 (1983).

T.D. Grekhova and L.N. El'nichnykh," Experimental Study of the Effectiveness of Saparal in Chronic Fluorine Intoxication", *Vopr. Gig. Prof. Patol. Tsveth. Chern. Metall.*, pp. 64-69 (1982).

Norio Shimamoto, et al., "Effects of 2,3-Dimethoxy-5methyl 6-(10'hydroxydecy)-1,4-benzoquine (cv2619) on the Energy Metabolism of Red Blood Cells of Rats", *Nippon Yakurigaku Zasshi*, Volume 80, pp. 137-145 (1984).

Steven L. Edwards, et al., "The Crystal Structure of Fluoride-inhibited Cytochrome c Peroxidase", *Journal of Biological Chemistry*, Volume 259, pp. 12984-12988 (1984).

Thomas L. Poulos, personal communication, 1985.

Z. Juzyszyn, "Chronic effect of ammonium fluoride on selected parameters of microsomal fracture of the rat liver with special reference to the cytochrome P-450 system", *Ann. Acad. Med. Stetin.*, Volume 37, pp. 49-64 (1991).

[The following is a list of studies showing not only that fluoride is not essential, but also that fluoride interferes with growth rate and reproduction.

T. Suzuki, "Effects of Low Fluoride Feeding Through Successive Generations on Rats", *Japanese Journal of Dental Health*, Volume 19, pp. 51-70 (1969).

G.W.A.E. Le Coultre-Mulder, et al., "Influence of the Fluorine Ion on the Growth in Vitro of Human amnion Cells, T-(Kidney) Cells, and Hela Cells", *Acta Physiologica et Pharmacologica Neerlandica*, Volume 15, pp. 1-19 (1969).

S. Tamura and K. Goto, "Experimental Study of Fluoride Toxicity", *Journal of Dental Research*, Volume 49, p. 672 (1970).

R.I. Byalik, "Effect of Various Concentrations of Fluorine and Manganese in the Drinking Water on the Tooth Enamel and Weight of Rats", *Nauch. Tr. Omsk. Med. Inst.*, Volume 69, pp. 35-37 (1966).

M.S. Sadilova and A.A. Petina, "The Hygienic Significance of Low Concentrations of Fluoride Entering the Organism by Various Routes of Administration", *Gigiena i Sanitariya*, Volume 35, pp. 14-17 (1970).

A.A. Petina and L.N. El'nichnykh, "Toxicological Characteristic of Fluorine During Its Simultaneous Entrance into an Organism Along with Drinking Water and Inhaled Air. II.", *Flyuoroz Ego Profil., Mater. Simp.*, 1967, pp. 153-163.

Chapter 14 The Second Fable: Fluoride Reduces Tooth Decay

Gerald Cox, "Causes and Control of Dental Caries", *Dental Rays*, Volume 13, pp. 14-18, 50-52 (1937).

Gerald Cox, "Discussion", *Journal of the American Medical Association*, Volume 113, p. 1753 (1938).

Wallace Armstrong and P.J. Brekhus, "Possible Relationship Between the Fluorine Content of Enamel and Resistance to Dental Caries", *Journal of Dental Research*, Volume 17, pp. 393-399 (1938).

Wallace Armstrong and Leon Singer, "Fluoride Contents of Enamel of Sound and Carious Human Teeth: A Reinvestigation", *Journal of Dental Research*, Volume 42, pp. 133-136 (1963).

Gerald Cox, et al., "Experimental Dental Caries IV. Fluorine and Its Relation to Dental Caries", *Journal of Dental Research*, Volume 18, pp. 481-490 (1939).

J.L. Hardwick and D.M. Bunting, "Effects of Fluoridation of Drinking Water or of a Cariogenic Diet on Caries Experience of Rats", *Journal of Dental Research*, Volume 50 (Supplement to No. 5), p. 1212 (1971).

Edward Sweeney, et al., "Effect of Alloxan Diabetes on Fluoride Retention and Caries Incidence in Rats", *Journal of Dental Research*, Volume 41, No. 4, pp. 866-874 (1962).

R. L. Spuller, et al., "The effect of low levels of sodium fluoride in drinking water on the incidence of dental caries in rats", *Caries Research*, Volume 20, pp. 556-558 (1986).

R. Spuller, et al., "Enhancement of dental caries by Coca Cola", *Journal of Dental Research (Special Issue/Abstracts)* , Volume 67, p. 318 (1988).

S. Beiraghi, et al., "Low level fluoride in drinking water and caries incidence in rats", *Journal of Dental Research (Special Issue/Abstracts)* , Volume 67, p. 318 (1988).

Hearings before a Subcommittee of the Committee on Appropriations, 96th Congress, Second Session Subcommittee on Labor-HEW, Pt. 3 (April 18,1980):1089-96

F.J. McClure and F.A. Arnold "Observations on induced dental caries in rats", *Journal of Dental Research*, Volume 20, pp. 97-105 (1941).

H. Trendley Dean, "Endemic Fluorosis and Its Relation to Dental Caries", *Public Health Reports*, Volume 53, pp. 1443-1452 (1938).

H. Trendley Dean, "Domestic Water and Dental Caries", *Public Health Reports*, Volume 57, pp. 1155-1179 (1942).

Fred Losee and Basel Bibby, "Carries Inhibition by Trace Elements Other than Fluoride", *New York State Dental Journal*, Volume 36, pp. 15-19 (1970).

T.G. Ludwig, et al., "Relationship of Concentrations of Eleven Elements in Public Water Supplies to Caries Prevalence in American Schoolchildren", *Australian Dental Journal*, Volume 15, pp. 126-132 (1970).

Eugene Zimmerman, "Oral Aspects of Excessive Fluorides in a Water Supply", *Journal of the American Dental Association*, Volume 50, pp. 272-277 (1955).

David Galagan, "Climate and Controlled Fluoridation", *Journal of the American Dental Association*, Volume 47, pp. 159-170 (1953).

Yoshitsugu Imai, "Relation Between Fluoride Concentration in Drinking Water and Dental Caries in Japan", *Koku Eisei Gakkai Zasshi*, Volume 22, No. 2, pp. 144-196 (1972).

Hearings Before a Subcommittee of the Committee on Appropriations, 96th Congress, Second Session Subcommittee on Labor-HEW, pp. 1089-1096 (April 18, 1980).

Personal Communications from J. Rogers, Chief Dental Officer, British Ministry of Health to John Yiamouyiannis, December 11, 1980.

H. Trendley Dean, et al., "Studies on Mass Control of Dental Caries Through Fluoridation of the Public Water supply", *Public Health Reports*, Volume 65, pp. 1403-1408 (1950).

"The Conduct of the Fluoridation Studies in the United Kingdom and the Results Achieved after Five Years", *Reports on Public Health and Medical Subjects No. 105*, British Ministry of Health, London, Her Majesty's Stationery Office, 1962, 50 pp.

"The Fluoridation Studies in the United Kingdom and the Results achieved after Eleven Years", *Reports on Public Health and Medical Subjects No. 122*, Department of Health and Social Security, Her Majesty's Stationery Office, 1969, 45pp.

J. Colquhoun, "Influence of Social Class and Fluoridation on Child Dental Health", *Community Dent Oral Epidemiol,*, Volume 13, pp. 37-41 (1985).

J. Colquhoun, "Child Dental Health Differences in New Zealand", *Community Health Studies*, Volume 11, pp. 85-90 (1987).

J. Colquhoun, "Fluoridation: Time for Reassessment", Submission to the Standing Committee on Social Policy of the Australian Capital Territory Legislative Assembly, Feb. 6, 1990.

J.A. Yiamouyiannis, "Water Fluoridation and Tooth Decay: Results from the 1986-1987 National Survey of U.S. Schoolchildren", *Fluoride* 1990; 23: 55-67.

R.M. Bell, et al., "Results of baseline dental exams in the national preventive dentistry demonstration program". R-2862-RWJ. Santa Monica, CA. Rand Corporation. 1982

A.S. Gray, "Fluoridation: Time for a New Baseline?" *Journal of the Canadian Dental Association,* Volume 53, pp. 763-765 (1987).

J.V. Kumar, et al., "Trends in Dental Fluorosis and Dental Caries Prevalences in Newburgh and Kingston, NY", *American Journal of Public Health,* Volume 79, pp. 565-569 (1989).

C.F. Hildebolt, et al., "Caries Prevalences among Geochemical Regions of Missouri", *American Journal of Physical Anthropology,* Volume 78, pp. 79-92, (1989).

R.L. Glass, "Secular Changes in Caries Prevalence in Two Massachusetts Towns", *Caries Research*, Volume 15, pp. 445-450 (1981).

T.M. McEniery and G.N. Davies, "Brisbane Dental Survey, 1977, A Comparative Study of Caries Experience of Children in Brisbane, Australia over a 20-Year Period", *Community Dentistry and Oral Epidemiology*, Volume 7, pp. 42-50 (1979).

P.B.V. Hunter, "The Prevalence of Dental Caries in 5-year-old New Zealand Children", *New Zealand Dental Journal*, Volume 75, pp. 154-157 (1979).

The Report of a Workshop on the Changes of Dental Caries Prevalence, British Association for the study of Community Health, 1981.

S.S. Krylov and K. Pemrolyd, "Deciduous tooth eruption and fluorosis in the case of increased fluorine content in the drinking water", *Stomatologiia,* (Mosk) Volume 61, pp. 75-77 (1982).

H.H. Neumann and N.A. DiSalvo, "Caries in the Otomi Indians of Mexico", *New York State Dental Journal*, Volume 24, pp. 63-68 (1956).

Kurt Rosenzweig, "Dentition of Bedouins in Israel: I. Epidemiology", *Journal of Dental Research,* Volume 47, No. 3, pp. 407-410 (1968).

A. Sheiham, "The Prevalence of Dental Caries in Nigerian Populations", *British Dental Journal*, Volume 123, pp. 144-148 (1967).

H. J. Mosha et al., "Changes in dental caries experience of 12-year olds in low fluoride urban and rural areas of Tanzania", *East Afr Med J.,* Volume 68, pp. 963-968 (1991).

D. Gaare, et al, "A Cross-Sectional Study of DMFT and CPITN scores in a group of Indonesian Soldiers", *Scandanavian Journal of Dental Research*, Volume 97, pp. 20-24 (1989).

T. Tijmstra, et al., "Effect of Socioeconomic Factors on the Observed Caries Reduction After Fluoride Tablet and Fluoride Toothpaste Consumption", *Community Dentistry and Oral Epidemiology*, Volume 6, pp. 227-230 (1978).

B. C. Stecksen, et al., "Dental Caries in Swedish 4-year-old Children. Changes between 1967 and 1987", *Swedish Dental Journal*, Volume 13, pp. 39-44 (1989).

A. J. Conti, et al., "A 3-Year Clinical Trial to Compare Efficacy of Dentifrices Containing 1.14% and .76% Sodium Monofluorophosphate", *Community Dentistry and Oral Epidemiology*, Volume 16, pp. 135-138 (1988).

K. H. Lu, et al., "A 3-Year Clinical comparison of a Sodium Monofluorophosphate Dentifrice with Sodium Fluoride Dentifrices in Children", *ASDC J Dent Child.*, Volume 54, pp. 241-244 (1987).

Goran Koch, et al., "Effect of 250 and 1000 ppm Fluoride Dentifrice on Caries", *Swedish Dental Journal*, Volume 6, pp. 233-238 (1982).

T. Cutress, et al., "Caries preventive effect of high fluoride and xylitol containing dentifrices", *ASDC J Dent Child.*, Volume 59, pp. 313-318 (1992).

J. E. Moorhead, et al., "The effect of supervised brushing on caries inhibition in school age children", *J. Clin. Dent*, Volume 2, pp. 97-102 (1991).

J. R. Mellberg, et al., "A study of the ability of an in situ remineralization model to differentiate between the effects of two fluoride dentifrices that produced significantly different clinical caries results", *Journal of Dental Research*, Volume 71, pp. 1169-1172 (1992).

Ola Haugejordan, et al., "An 11-Year Follow-Up Study of Dental Caries After Discontinuation of School-Based Fluoride Programs", *Acta Odontol Scand*, Volume 48, pp. 257-263 (1990).

J. A. Disney, et al., "Comparative Effects of a 4-year Mouthrinse Program on High and Low Caries Forming Grade 1 Children", *Community Dentistry and Oral Epidemiology*, Volume 17, pp. 46-56 (1989).

J. A. Disney, et al., "A Case Study in Testing the Conventional Wisdom: School-Based Fluoride Mouthrinse Programs in the USA", *Community Dentistry and Oral Epidemiology*, Volume 18, pp. 46-56 (1990).

"Preventing Tooth Decay: Results from a Four-Year National Study", Robert Wood Johnson Foundation, Special Report Number 2/1983, 18pp.

Anna-Karin Holm and Roland Anderson, "Enamel mineralization disturbance in children with known early exposure to fluorides", *Community Dentistry and Oral Epidemiology*, Volume 10, pp. 335-339 (1982).

K.W. Stephen et al., "Incisor enamel mottling prevalence in child cohorts which had or had not taken fluoride supplements from 0-12 years of age", *Proc Finn Dent Soc*, Volume 87, pp. 595-605 (1991)

H. Kalsbeek, et al., "Dental fluorosis in relation to the use of fluoride tablets", *Ned Tijdschr Tandleelkd*, Volume 97, pp. 269-273 (1990).

H. Kalsbeek, "Use of fluoride tablets and effect on prevalence of dental caries and dental fluorosis", *Community Dentistry and Oral Epidemiology*, Volume 20, pp. 241-245 (1992).

M.J. Larsen et al., "Dental fluorosis among participants in a non supervised fluoride tablet program", *Community Dentistry and Oral Epidemiology*, Volume 17, pp. 204-206 (1989).

Jan Widenheim, et al., "Preeruptive effect of sodium fluoride tablets on caries in children from twelve to seventeen years of age", *Community Dentistry and Oral Epidemiology*, Volume 14, pp. 1-4 (1986).

K.W. Stephen et al., "Combined Fluoride therapies. A 6-year double-blind school-based preventive dentistry study in Inverness Scotland", *Community Dentistry and Oral Epidemiology*, Volume 18, pp. 244-248 (1990).

J. Widenheim and D. Birkhed, "Caries-preventive effect on primary and permanent teeth and cost-effectiveness of an NaF tablet preschool program", *Community Dentistry and Oral Epidemiology*, Volume 19, pp. 88-92 (1991).

Chapter 15 See How They Pollute

Alcoa Advertisement from the *Journal of the American Water Works Association*, Volume 43, No. 6 (1960).

"An Island Unfit for Man or Beast", *Maclean's*, July 30, 1979, pp. 40-41.

"Industrial Fluoride Pollution, Chronic Fluoride Poisoning in Cornwall Island Cattle", *The Cornell Veterinarian*, Volume 69 (Supplement 8) 1979, 70 pp.

"Sick Cows, Human Fears in Maryland County", *The Washington Post*, August 7, 1977.

"Tons of Fluoride Emitted in 3 Florida Counties", *Sarasota Herald Tribune*, August 14, 1977.

F.F.V. Atkinson and Gordon Hard, "Chronic Fluorosis in the Guinea-pig", *Nature*, Volume 211, No. 5047, pp. 429-430 (1966).

Donald Hillman, et al., "Hypothyroidism and Anemia Related to Fluoride in Dairy Cattle", *Journal of Dairy Science*, Volume 62, pp. 416-423 (1979).

"Dairy Feed is Called Dangerous", *Detroit Free Press*, September 30, 1977.

"Dog Ailments May be Tied to Pet Foods", *The Grand Rapids Press*, August 14, 1981.

Chapter 16 The Conspiracy: Early History

"Editorial: Chronic Fluorine Intoxication", *Journal of American Medical Association*, Volume 123, p. 150 (1943)

"Editorial: Effect of Fluorine on Dental Caries", *Journal of American Dental Association*, Volume 31, pp. 1360-1363 (1944).

Compare this editorial with a more recent statement made by the American Dental Association in the March 24, 1980 issue of ADA News, in response to Environmental Protection Agency regulations requiring defluoridation of water supplies with fluoride contents above 2.4 parts per million. The ADA stated that *"there is no evidence implicating naturally occurring fluorides as a health hazard even at eight (parts per million). . . The ADA recognizes that fluorosis may occur as a result of ingesting high concentrations of fluoride, . . . however, it does not agree that tooth mottling itself damages teeth or poses a health hazard."* To see exactly what fluoride does to teeth and the damage to the biological processes that is necessary to occur before teeth are mottled, see Chapter 5. The real reason the American Dental Association is opposing the defluoridation regulations set out by the Environmental Protection Agency is quite clear from their own admission, in the same issue of the ADA News: *"The ADA . . . opposes the EPA regulation because of concern that the labeling of excess fluoride as a contaminant will undermine the efforts of the dental profession and government in promoting fluoridation of community water supplies."*

Dr. R. McNeil, "The Fight For Fluoridation", *Oxford University Press*, 1957, p. 50.

Hearings before the Committee on Interstate and Foreign Commerce, House of Representatives, Eighty-third Congress, Second Session on H.R. 2341, May 25-27, 1954, p. 51.

Joel Griffiths, "Fluoride: Commie Plot or Capitalist Ploy", *Covert Action*, Number 24, pp. 26-29, 63-66 (1992).

Proceedings of the Fourth Annual Conference of State Dental Directors with the Public Health Service and the Children's Bureau, Federal Security Building, Washington, D.C., June 6-8, 1951.

A.L. Miller, "Fluoridation of Water- Extension of Remarks", *Congressional Record*, March 25, 1952, pp. A1899-A1901.

Comments on Opponents of Fluoridation. *Journal of the American Dental Association*, Volume 71, p. 1155-1183 (1965).

Chapter 17

The Conspiracy: The Second Generation 1965-1993

Russell Rowlett, Confidential Memorandum Regarding John Yiamouyiannis—Antifluoridation Talks, August 11, 1970.

Russell Rowlett, Letter to John Small, August 10, 1970.

Yiamouyiannis J. "How Eighteen Federal and State Health Department Employees Conspired to Cover up the Hazards of Fluoridation Documented", December 28, 1989

E. G. Knox, et al., "Fluoridation and the prevalence of congenital malformations", *Community Medicine*, Volume 2, pages 190-194 (1980).

J. D. Erickson, "Down's syndrome, water fluoridation, and maternal age", *Teratology*, Volume 21, pages 177-180 (1980).

J. W. Knutson, "An evaluation of the Grand Rapids Water Fluoridation Project", *Journal of the Michigan Medical Society*, Volume 53, pages 1001-1006 (1954).

Rogot, E., et al., "Trends in urban mortality in relation to fluoridation status", *American Journal of Epidemiology*, Volume 107, pages 104-112 (1978).

Transcript of May 11,1978 testimony of Leo Kinlen in the case of Aikenhead v. Borough of West View, No. GD 4585-78, Court of Common Pleas of Allegheny County, Pennsylvania, pages 29-30.

Transcript of the testimony of Richard Doll from The Scottish Court Case, pages 19260-19261.

Chapter 18   The Conspiracy: Containing the Cancer Link

"The National Cancer Program (Part 2 - Fluoridation of Public Drinking Water)", *Hearings Before a Subcommittee of the Committee on Government Operations*, House of Representatives, 95th Congress First Session, September 21 and October 12, 1977 p. 239.

"The National Cancer Program (Part 2 - Fluoridation of Public Drinking Water)", *Hearings Before a Subcommittee of the Committee on Government Operations*, House of Representatives, 95th Congress First Session, September 21 and October 12, 1977, 580 pp.

June 18, 1976

Dr. Leo Kinlen
Department of Regius Dept. of Medicine
Oxford University, Radcliffe Infirmary
Oxford, England

Dear Dr. Kinlen,

Thank you for your letter concerning our reanalysis of the Burk and Yiamouyiannis time-trend study of fluoridation. Indeed, Drs. Burk and Yiamouyiannis have tried to make an issue of the fact that they have not seen the "actual data" leading to our reanalysis. I am quite unsympathetic to these objections, since we purposefully used only published data in doing the reanalysis, so we could not be accused of concealing data. Therefore, all that is necessary for anyone in this country to check our analyses is to be aware of basic principles of biostatistics and epidemiology, and have a public library card. I recognize, however, that this same case of access to the relevant data does not exist for people in other countries. I have therefore enclosed the relevant numbers for 1950, 1960, and 1970, that led to our adjustments. The numbers of residents, grouped by age according to the age-grouping for the rates used, are all taken from the routine publications of the Bureau of the Census. The numbers of deaths come from the routine publications of the National Center for Health Statistics. The age and race-specific mortality rates for cancer come from the 1950 vital statistics volume published by the National Center for Health Statistics. The rates are given for those under one year of age and for those from one to 4 years of age. From the published data we recalculated rates for the entire zero to four age group in order to apply these to the populations we had. These recalculated rates are written in the margin of the copy of the table containing the rates. Using these numbers, you should hopefully be able to reproduce our SMR's. We also calculated SMR's for 1955 and 1965, deriving the intercensal populations by linear interpolation. These SMR's are not essential for the reanalysis. However, if you wish to recalculate them also, I can send you the observed number of deaths in these two years for the relevant cities. Please let me know if you reach any different conclusion than we have by using these data. If you are queried as to how you obtained the data, I would appreciate it if you would indicate that all of the raw data are available from routine publications available to anyone.

I hope this information is useful to you.

Sincerely yours,

Robert N. Hoover, M.D.

13 July 1976

Dr. Robert Hoover
Dept. Of Health, Education and Welfare
Public Health Service, National Institutes of Health
Bethesda, Maryland 20014

Dear Bob,

Thank you very much for your letter of 18 June, and for the details of
the data used in the re-analysis of the material used by Burk et al. I
take your point about the raw data being available in routine publications which are easy of access, at least in the US., and we will stress
this.

Because of criticism which the Royal College has received over the
question of cancer and fluoride, the Royal Statistical Society has been
asked for an independent opinion. Scientifically this would ordinarily
not have been justified, but politically it was felt that our position
should be seen to be unassailable.

If the final version of your paper on the subject differs from the
version which you kindly sent us, we would be most grateful if we
could receive a copy. We are always months behind in receiving the
Journal of the NCI - perhaps because our copies come by surface mail.

With best wishes,

Yours sincerely,

Leo Kinlen
University of Oxford
Department of the Regius Professor of Medicine
Radcliffe Infirmary
Oxford OX2 GHE

28th April 1977

Professor D.J. Newell, Ph.D.
Dept. Of Medical Statistics
21 Claremont Place,
The University of Newcastle Upon Tyne NE2 4AA

Dear David,

I have succeeded in my self-imposed task of being able to claim that I have verified for myself the data we relied upon. The OPCS library provided everything necessary - piles of State volumes for the 1950 and 1970 censuses - and I was able to add up the deaths, see the page giving national cancer death rates, and find the population figures for every city. It was not possible to transcribe and/or add these latter up because of the scale of the problem - 17 five-year age-groups, 4 races or places of origin (native-born white, foreign born ditto, negro, other) and the sexes. Moreover the exact definition of each city required more knowledge than I had - each tended to have three or four sub-regions, and the total was clearly too large to be the right figure. However I now feel much easier in my mind, in that it clearly was physically possible to do what Hoover claimed anyone could do, and we cannot be accused of having access to figures Burk and Yiamouyiannis could not get at.

I even found a mistake - the total number of cancer deaths in Boston in 1970 was not 1667, but 1452. The former figure was for Suffolk county. Thus the crude death rate for non-fluoridated cities would appear to be not 197.16 but 194.24. On the other hand, perhaps Suffolk County is the proper population called Boston (though in every other city the figure given is for the city itself). If there are no compensating errors, the effect of this is to make the excess cancer-rate in the non-fluoridated cities to have increased by just the same proportion as in the fluoridated.

Ah well, I should have left well alone, no doubt.

Yours,

P.D. Oldham, M.A., D.Sc.
Medical Research Council
Llandough Hospital
Penarth, Glamorgan CF6 1XW

September 26, 1977

Dr. Leo Kinlen
University of Oxford
Dept. of the Regius Professor of Medicine
Radcliffe Infirmary
Oxford OX2 6HE ENGLAND

As I am sure you are aware by this time, the National Health Federation
has recently found an error in our tabulation of total number of 1970
observed cancer deaths for the "non-fluoridated" cities in our reanalysis of
the NHF time trend study. The error was of a trivial magnitude and does
not change the conclusions of either our reanalysis or yours in the Lancet.
Instead of 14,487 deaths in the non-fluoridated cities in 1970 the number
should be 14,272. The error arose not from arithmetic but from geography.
Specifically, when we tabulated deaths in the city of Boston. We included
all of Suffolk county rather than just the city of Boston. Therefore, Boston
deaths in 1970 should read 1,452, rather than 1,667 as I transmitted to you
in June of 1976. We have checked and rechecked the numbers of deaths
and the populations in 1950 and 1970. In doing this, we discovered several
minor errors in the populations also. As it turns out, none of the errors
lead to any differences in the SMR's calculated. However, I am enclosing a
copy of the page of populations that I sent you in June of last year with the
incorrect numbers crossed out and the correct numbers written in. You
will note that, in fact, the largest error tends to work in favor of the NHF
position, confirming my opinion that the errors made were random. As I
have mentioned, incorporating the correct figures does not change our
conclusions, and I believe it does not change yours either. Specifically, the
SMR for the non-fluoridated cities based on the 1950 rates becomes 1.17,
instead of 1.19 as we had in our original analysis. This means that the
SMR rose by 1% in the fluoridated areas (1.23 to 1.24) while at the same
time rising 2% in the non-fluoridated areas (1.15 to 1.17).

I am sorry for this error, particularly since it seems to have been perpetuated by yourselves and the Royal Statistical Society. I am a bit distressed
also that neither you nor the Society checked some of the original numbers.
When Professor Doll visited us, I believe I suggested that the numbers be
checked against the original sources, since our reanalysis were done very
hastily and under severe political pressure. In fact, I thought the Society
had abstracted that data themselves, since I did not send them any of the
original material. However, they must have obtained it elsewhere, as they
have the erroneous number also. I am writing Dr. Newell and enclosing a
copy of this letter so that he will be kept informed.

While none of the conclusions change, the anti-fluoridationists are certainly
having a grand time with this error. They are claiming that we are
responsible for creating an "international embarrassment." If indeed it has
caused such for you, Sir Richard, or the Royal Statistical Society, I sincerely apologize.

It is regrettable that the NHF seems to be able to divert attention from good, solid, negative studies such as yours and ours, to their own "study" which didn't even adjust for race or age. Even if a slight difference in the direction they hypothesized had appeared in their data, the overwhelming weight of evidence from other, better controlled studies would be negative. Somehow this gets lost in the rhetoric.

We are now in the process of checking the numbers for 1960, 1955, and 1965, and calculating SMR's for all of the others years for which data are available. We have also calculated (and checked) SMR's for 1950 and 1970 for each of the individual cities. This table is enclosed for your information, and yields the same conclusion as does the aggregated data.

If it helps you at all in your discussions, you should know that Dr. Taves did in fact abstract the original data for his analyses by himself from his own library. Therefore, his conclusions, which were the same as ours, were based on a completely independent assessment of the data as well as the analyses.

I am in the process of writing a letter to the Lancet which will correct our error and point out that it does not change our conclusions. I will also take this opportunity to correct some erroneous statements made by Dr. Yiamouyiannis in his recent letter to the Lancet. Specifically, I will point out that while the total age distribution may not have shifted dramatically, the shift to an older population in the fluoridated cities was marked among "white", emphasizing the need for simultaneous control of race and age. In addition, he states that the increase in cancer mortality rate among non-whites is attributable to increased urbanization and is therefore not present in central cities in this country. This is, of course, false. The increase occurs absolutely everywhere (in every region and every urban and rural location) in this country where "non-white" indicated predominantly black population.

Again, my apologies for the error and any embarrassment it has caused you. There is no excuse for it. Yet if an error of 200 deaths on the base of 14,000 is the most serious criticism of all of our fluoride-related activities over the past two years, in the presence of the pressure and the urgency under which we were working, then I think my staff actually deserves some sort of award.

Sincerely yours,

Robert N. Hoover, M.D.

Head, Environmental Studies Section
Environmental Epidemiology Branch
RNH/gca

cc: Richard Doll

10th October 1977

Dr. R.N. Hoover,
Head, Environmental Studies Section,
Environmental Epidemiology Branch
Department of Health, Education and Welfare,
Public Health Service

National Institutes of Health,
Bethesda, Maryland 20014
UNITED STATES OF AMERICA

Dear Dr. Hoover,
                        Fluoridation and Cancer

Thank you for sending me a copy of your letter to Leo Kinlen.

The position that we took with your data appears on p. 134 of our paper in Applied Statistics. I quote:

"The data . . . were extracted from the routine publications of the US Bureau of the Census and accumulated by the National Cancer Institute. We have no reason to doubt their ability to add and tabulate these numbers."

At the time that our paper was going to press, Peter Oldham felt he should reassure himself that the National Health Federation was wrong in its statement that the data were not available. He went to the Office of Population Censuses and Surveys in London, with the result shown in his enclosed letter dated 28th April. Rightly or wrongly, I suggested, and he agreed, that we should not delay publication any further. This would have involved us in trying to clarify your demographic conventions, and then recalculating the tables throughout: as the paper was already past the final proof stage, it would have caused considerable disturbance in the Editorial office either to delete and postpone the paper, or to have held the whole edition which was already later than planned. The conclusions would not have been changed.

If it will give you any consolation, I also enclose a copy of my letter dated 10th June to Dr. Burk, which so far has produced no response at all in correcting their paper now published in Fluoride, Vol. 10, No. 3, 1977, 102-123.

Yours sincerely,

David Newell
The University of Newcastle Upon Tyne
Department of Medical Statistics
21 Claremont Place NE2 4AA

[The following is an excerpt written by John Yiamouyiannis and published in the January 21, 1978 issue of The Lancet.]

"On June 18, 1976, Dr. Robert N. Hoover sent the National Cancer Institute data on cancer mortality and fluoridation to Dr. L.J. Kinlen. In the accompanying letter he writes: 'If you are queried as to how you obtained the data, I would appreciate if you would indicate that all of the raw data are available from routine publications available to anyone.' Doll and Kinlen did just that. They used the N.C.I.'s figures without alteration and claimed that they obtained their data from 'routine publications'. Unfortunately for Doll and Kinlen, the N.C.I. made a serious mathematical or tabulation error which was repeated in their paper.

The errors in the N.C.I./Doll-Kinlen data were discovered by Dr. Dean Burk and myself and transmitted to the Lancet on September 5, 1977 and to the N.C.I. shortly before the Congressional hearing in September/October investigation of an alleged cover-up of the fluoridation-cancer link. Dr. Hoover admitted the error and its duplication on September 26, 1977, in a letter to Dr. Kinlen in which he wrote: 'I am sorry for this error, particularly since it seems to have been perpetuated by yourselves and the Royal Statistical Society.' Dr. P.D. Oldham uncovered N.C.I.'s error, yet in his paper for the R.S.S. with Prof. D.J. Newell, he used the erroneous data.

"More important that the mathematical errors passed on by the N.C.I. (which account for about 3500 cancer deaths a year) are the methodological errors that were also spoon-fed to Oldham and Newell and Doll and Kinlen by the N.C.I. (and which account for about 9000 cancer deaths per year). These include omission of 90-95% of the data available and the selection as one of their data points a year (1970) during which fluoridation of the control group had already started."

"The National Cancer Program (Part 2—Fluoridation of Public Drinking Water)", Hearings Before a Subcommittee of the Committee on Government Operations, House of Representatives, 95th Congress First Session, September 21 and October 12, 1977, pp. 233, 501.

Arthur Upton, Letter to John Yiamouyiannis, January 31, 1978.

J.K. Maurer, et al. "Two-year carcinogenicity study of sodium fluoride in rats", *Journal of the National Cancer Institute*; 82: 1118-1126 (1990).

Procter and Gamble. "Carcinogenicity studies with sodium fluoride", Presented at the National Institute of Environmental Health Sciences July 27, 1985).

Bucher JR, Hejtmancik MR, Toft JD, Persing RL, Eustis SL, Haseman JK. Interpretation and Conclusions of the National Toxicology Program's Rodent Carcinogenicity Studies with Sodium Fluoride, 1990, 14pp.

S.E. Hrudey et al., "Drinking Water Fluoridation and Osteosarcoma", *Can J Pub Health,* Volume 81, pp. 415-416 (1990).

S. M. McGuire et al., "Is There a Link Between Fluoridated Water and Osteosarcoma?", *Journal of the American Association* , Volume 122, pp. 39-45 (1991).

R. N. Hoover et al., "Time Trends for Bone and Joint Cancers and Osteosarcomas in the Surveillance, Epidemiology and End Results (SEER) Program." In: *Review of Fluoride: Benefits and Risks*. Report of the Ad Hoc Committee on Fluoride of the Committee to Coordinate Environmental Health and Related Programs, United States Public Health Service, DHHS, 1991 Feb: F1-F7

P. D. Cohn, "A Brief Report on the Association of Drinking Water Fluoridation and the Incidence of Osteosarcoma among Young Males", *New Jersey Department of Health*, Trenton, NJ, 1992 Nov

M. C. Mahoney et al., "Bone Cancer Incidence Rates in New York", *Amer J Pub Health,* Volume 81, pp. 81:475 (1991).

S.C. Freni and DW Gaylor, "International Trends in the Incidence of Bone Cancer are not Related to Drinking Water Fluoridation", *Cancer* , Volume 70, pp. 70:611-618 (1992).

Richard Doll and Leo Kinlen, "Fluoridation of Water and Cancer Mortality in the U.S.A.", *Lancet*, pp. 1300-1332 (June 1977).

D.J. Newell, "Fluoridation of Water Supplies and Cancer - A Possible Association?" *Applied Statistics*, Volume 26, No. 2, pp. 125-135 (1977).

J. A. Disney, et al., "A Case Study in Testing the Conventional Wisdom: School-Based Fluoride Mouthrinse Programs in the USA", *Community Dentistry and Oral Epidemiology*, Volume 18, pp. 46-56 (1990).

A. Taylor, "Sodium Fluoride in the Drinking Water of Mice", *Dental Digest*, Volume 60, pp. 170-172 (1954).

Irwin Herskowitz and Isabel Norton, "Increased Incidence of Melanotic Tumors in Two Strains of Drosphila Melanogaster Following Treatment with Sodium Fluoride", *Genetics*, Volume 48, pp. 307-310 (1963).

A. Taylor and N.C. Taylor "Effect of Fluoride on Tumor Growth", *Proceedings of the Society of Experimental Biology and Medicine* , Volume 65, pp. 252-255 (1965).

Chapter 19   The Extended Conspiracy: Their Evil Network

"OSHA Firing Attempt Called Scientific Muffling", *Chemical & Engineering News*, Volume 59, No. 30, pp. 29-30 (July 27, 1981).

Frank Greve, "Deletion in Benzene-Cancer Study stirs Controversy", *The Houston Post*, August 8, 1982 [A more complete account of this affair is given in the journal, Science, Volume 217, pp. 914-915 (1982); in a press release from congressman David Obey's office, dated October 1, 1982, he pointed out that the further funding for international programs for the study of toxic chemicals has been taken away from the National Cancer Institute.]

Joseph Botta, "Fluoridation the Cancer Scare", *Consumer Reports*, Volume 43, No. 7, pp. 392-396 (1978).

Joseph Botta, "Six Ways to Mislead the Public"," *Consumer Reports*, Volume 43, No. 8, pp. 480-482 (1978).

Stephen Barrett, "Fluoridation: Poison-Mongers Delaying Health for Millions?" *Journal of American Dental Association*, Volume 93, p. 880 (1976).

Stephen Barrett, Letter to Mrs. N. Johnson of Brainerd, Minnesota, March 8, 1972

Stephen Barrett, Letter to Mike Liptak of Brainerd, Minnesota, April 4, 1972.

Stephen Barrett, Letter to Mary Bernhardt, Secretary, Council of Health, American Dental Association, Chicago, Illinois, May 12, 1972.

Stephen Barrett, Mary Bernhardt, et al., *Health Robbers*, George F. Stickley Co., Philadelphia, 1976.

Stephen Barrett, Letter to Alexis Bell, President, Faculty Club, University of California, Berkeley, October 1, 1975.

Thomas Jukes, Letter to E.C. Walters, Faculty Club, University of California, Berkeley, September 29, 1975.

Thomas Jukes, Letter to Alexis Bell, President, Faculty Club, University of California, Berkeley, October 3, 1975.

Thomas Jukes, To Members of the Faculty Club, Board of Directors, University of California, Berkeley, October 8, 1975.

Warren Winklestein, Letter to Professor Alexis Bell, University of California, Berkeley, October 14, 1975.

E.L.R. Stokstad, Letter to Professor Alexis Bell, University of California, Berkeley, October 21, 1975.

Stephen Barrett, Letter to the National News Council, New York, May 31, 1977.

Joel Boriskin, Letter to the National News Council, New York, June 24, 1977.

William Jarvis, Letter to the National Enquirer, Lantana, Florida, April 22, 1977.

Peter Petrakis, "Some Fluoridationists Don't Believe in Academic Freedom", *Health Action*, Volume 2, No. 2, pp. 11-19 (1981).

Eugene Rogot, et al., "Trends in urban mortality in relation to fluoridation status", *American Journal of Epidemiology*, volume 107, pages 104-112 (1978).

G.R. Martin, et al., "Lack of Cytogenetic Effects on Mice or Mutations in Salmonella Receiving Sodium Fluoride", *Mutation Research* 66: 159-167 (1979).

Chapter 21 Good News

Kevin Oliver, Master Thesis, University of Kansas, Lawrence, Kansas, 1983.

Index

A

abdomen 137

abdominal pain 9-11, 14

Abishev, Kh A. 37

abnormal lung function 12

abnormalities in brain
 tissue 70

Abuse of the Scientific Literature in an Antifluoridation
 Pamphlet 155-158, 187

acetyl-CoA synthetase 93

acetylcholinesterase 92,
 97, 175

aching bones 7, 24

acid glycerol phosphatase 92

acid phosphatase 93

acne 20

Acquaviva Platani 3

Acute Fluoride Poisoning 13

ADA, see American Dental
 Association

Adamson, Richard 167, 184

adrenalin 18

advertising 143

age, race, and sex 78, 79, 82,
 89, 166, 178

aging 3, 5, 6, 24, 25, 26,
 31, 32, 33, 38, 39, 52,
 53, 60, 63, 91
 of the bones 56

air pollution 13, 136

airborne fluorides 12, 13, 52,
 108, 133

Akron (Ohio) Regional Poison
 Center 13

Aksyuk, A.F. 56

Albright, J.A. 53

ALCOA, see Aluminum Com-
 pany of America

alkaline pyrophosphatase 92

Allegany, MD 127

Allen, TX 128

allergens 8

allergic or allergic-type
 responses 8, 27, 97, 99, 201

Alliance, OH 127

Allman, D.W. 29

Allukian, Myron 153

Alpine, OR 128

altered data 167

Alton, IL 127

aluminum 11, 12, 13, 29,
 61, 105, 133-138, 141, 185

Aluminum Company of
 America 41, 114, 134,
 140-2, 147, 185

Amarillo, TX 42

ameloblastic squamous cell
 dysplasias 85

ameloblasts
 35, 37, 40, 45, 46, 47
 precancerous 85

American Chemical Society
 206

American Council of Science
 and Health 153, 169, 187

American Dental Association
 134, 135, 140-160, 167,
 172, 181, 184, 186, 187,
 190, 191

American Medical Associa-
 tion 141, 147, 186, 187

American Oral Health Institute 155

amides 94, 96

amino acids 35, 94, 95

Amsterdam 104

anaphylactic 24

Anderson, Jack 205

Chemical Abstracts Service
150
chemical industry 153, 169
Chemical Industry Institute of
Technology 168
Chemical Manufacturers
Association 184
chemicals 32
chemotactic response 27
Chen, S. 37
Cherry Creek, CO 127
Chicago, IL 74, 81
Chicopee, MA 128
Chief Dental Officer 157
childhood diseases 21
chin 137
China 41
chondroblasts 35, 47
chondromas 170
chordoma 170
Chowchilla, CA 128
Christchurch 125, 131
chromosome damage 64-70,
197, 198; see also genetic
damage
chromosomes 62, 98
chronic fluoride poisoning
135, 148, 201
Cicero 149
Cincinnati, OH 74, 203
Cisneros, Henry 194
citrullinase 93
Clark, Robert 31
Clarke, David 206, 208
Clarksville, IN 127
clay 105, 138
Cleveland, OH 74, 81, 127,
203
Clinton, Indiana 203
Cloverdale, OR 127
Clovis, NM 42
coal miners 105

coal-burning power 138, 185
Coca Cola 101, 118
coffee 100, 105
Cohen 17
Cohn, Perry 171
Coldspring, TX 127
Colgate-Palmolive 207
collagen 5, 24, 34-40, 46,
47, 56-58, 60, 61
breakdown 25
metabolism 38
mineralization 39
synthesis 36, 37, 39, 47
Collins, James 152, 155
Colorado Brown Stain 3, 41
Colorado Springs, CO 42, 119
Colquhoun, John 43, 125,
149, 178, 206
Columbus 75
coma 18, 20
comprehensive list of localities
with fluoride 100
Concordia Co., LA 129
Condon, Louis 202
Conejo, CA 128
congenital malformations 161
Congress 166, 170
Congressional hearings 142,
200
Congressional Record
142, 165
Conibear, Shirley 12
Cons, Naham 19
conspiracy 140-200, 202,
208
Constipation 7
Consumer Reports 186,
187, 201, 203
control of protein and enzyme
synthesis 62
convulsions 18
Conway, SC 42

rivers   133, 141
Rivkin   29
RNA   63, 91
Robin, J.C.   54
Rocky Mountain Poison Center   14
rodenticide   103, 113, 134
Rogot, Eugene   195
Roholm, Kaj   13
Rolling Rock   101
Rorki   50
Rovin, Sheldon   13, 153
Rowe, David   160, 161
Royal College of Physicians   166, 201
Royal Statistical Society   166, 201
Ruckelshaus, William   158
Russia   12

S

Sack, W.H.   143
safe   201, 207
Safe Water Foundation   4, 210
Saideke   50
saliva   7
Salt Lake City   93
San Antonio, TX   81, 127, 194, 195
San Diego, CA   81
San Francisco, CA   75, 81, 93, 128
Sandstead, A.A.   109
sarcoma   4, 170
Saunders, Milton   19, 20
Schlegel, H.H.   13
Schneiderman, Marvin   165, 180, 201, 203
Schnitzler, C.M.   55
school rinse programs   22
schools   103

Schour, Isaac   44, 45
Schwarz, Klaus   108, 109
science   148, 187
scleroderma   60, 61
Scotland   195
scotomas   11
Seattle, WA   74, 81, 84
seeds   101
Segretto, V.A.   42, 179
seizure   19
Sencer, David   182
senility   3, 61
shallow breathing   7
Shamokin, PA   127
Sharma, Y.D.   37
Sharrett, A. R.   195
Shea, John   9
sheep   2
shin splints   57
shoulder tendinitis   57
Shupe, James   88, 160
side-effects   7
silver/mercury amalgam fillings   181
Singer, Leon   109
Singh, A.   48, 51, 60
skeletal and dental fluorosis   10
skeletal disorders   205
skeletal fluorosis   4, 50, 51, 53, 100, 159, 179
skin   1, 4, 5, 7, 8, 10, 26, 32, 35, 37, 38, 39, 58, 60, 61
  diseases   24
  eruptions   8, 9
  problems   25
  rash   7, 26, 32
  reaction   97
skinny   135
slander   148, 157, 186, 203
slobbering   137

PARADISE NATURAL FOODS
1868 N. Hillfield Rd. #9
Layton, Utah 84041
(801) 773-3529